A TREATISE ON THE Theory and Practice OF MIDWIFERY.

By W. SMELLIE, M. D.

LONDON:
Printed for D. Wilson, at Plato's Head, near Round-Court, in the Strand.
MDCCLII.

This facsimile printing of the First Edition
of A Treatise on the Theory and Practice of Midwifery
was made in 1974 by Scolar Press
39 Great Russell Street, London, and Ilkley, Yorkshire
and bound by Newdigate Press, Dorking
for Baillière Tindall, London, a division of Cassell and
Collier Macmillan Publishers Ltd
and Robert E. Krieger Publishing Co. Inc., New York
on the occasion of the
Twentieth British Congress of Obstetrics and Gynaecology
London, July 1974

ISBN 0 7020 0522 3 (Baillière Tindall, London)
0 88275 159 X (Robert E. Krieger, New York)

PREFACE.

I At first intended to have publish-ed this treatise in different lec-tures, as they were delivered in one course of Midwifery; but I found that method would not answer so well, in a work of this kind, as in teaching: because in the course of my lectures, almost every observation has a reference to the working of those machines which I have contri-ved to resemble and represent real women and children; and on which all the kinds of different labours are demonstrated, and even performed by every individual student.

I have, therefore, divided the whole into an Introduction, and four Books, distinguished by Chapters, Sections, and Numbers; and have industriously avoided all theory, except so much as may ſerve to whet the genius of young practitioners, and be as hints to introduce more valuable diſcoveries in the art.

The Introduction contains a ſummary account of the practice of Midwifery, both among the ancients and moderns, with the improvements which have been hitherto made in it; and this I have exhibited for the information of thoſe who have not had time or opportunity to peruſe the books from which it is collected; that by ſeeing at once the whole extent of the art, they may be the more able to judge for themſelves, and regulate their practice by thoſe authors who have written moſt judiciouſly upon the ſubject. The knowledge of theſe things will alſo help to raiſe a laudable ſpirit of emulation, that never fails to promote uſeful enquiries, which often redound to the honour of art, as well as to the advantage of ſociety.

Though

Though I have endeavoured to treat every thing in the moſt diſtinct and conciſe manner, perhaps many directions that may occur in the third Book, may be thought too minute and trivial by thoſe who have already had the advantage of an extenſive practice; but the work being principally undertaken with a view to refreſh the memory of thoſe who have attended me, and for the inſtruction of young practitioners in general, I thought it was neceſſary to mention every thing that might be uſeful in the courſe of practice.

At firſt, my deſign was to have inſerted caſes, by way of illuſtration, according to the method of *La Motte*; but, upon further deliberation, I thought ſuch a plan would too much embarraſs the ſtudent in the progreſs of his reading: and therefore I have reſolved, in imitation of *Mauriceau*, to publiſh a ſecond volume of hiſtories, digeſted into a certain number of claſſes or collections, with proper references to the particular parts of this treatiſe; ſo that the reader, when he wants to ſee the illuſtration, may turn over to it at his leiſure, according to the directions that ſhall be laid down.

Thoſe claſſes will conſiſt of the moſt uſeful caſes and obſervations, partly culled from the moſt approved authors, but chiefly collected from my own practice, and that of my correſpondents and former pupils, by whom I have been conſulted.

Nor will the reader, I hope, imagine, that ſuch a fund will be inſufficient for the purpoſe; or that this treatiſe is cooked up in a hurry, when I inform him, that above ſix years ago I began to commit my lectures to paper, for publication: and from that period, have from time to time altered, amended, and digeſted what I had written, according to the new

lights

lights I received from ſtudy and experience. Neither did I pretend to teach Midwifery, till after I had practiſed it ſucceſsfully for a long time in the country; and the obſervations I now publiſh, are the fruits not only of that opportunity, but more immediately of my practice in *London*, during ten years, in which I have given upwards of two hundred and eighty courſes of Midwifery, for the inſtruction of more than nine hundred pupils, excluſive of female ſtudents: and in that ſeries of courſes, one thouſand one hundred and fifty poor women have been delivered in preſence of thoſe who attended me; and ſupported during their lying-in, by the ſtated collection of my pupils: over and above thoſe difficult caſes to which we were often called by midwives, for the relief of the indigent.

Theſe conſiderations, together with that of my own private practice, which hath been pretty extenſive, will, I hope, ſcreen me from the imputation of arrogance, with regard to the task I have undertaken; and I flatter myſelf, that the Performance will not be unſerviceable to mankind.

It was my intention to inſert in this Compendium, plates of the moſt uſeful inſtruments appertaining to the art of Midwifery; but as large drawings could not be properly bound in a book of ſo ſmall a ſize, I have reſolved to publiſh them in folio, with that ſet of prints which I am now preparing, according to the propoſals ſpecified in the advertiſement at the end of this volume: mean while, the inſtruments themſelves which I principally uſe and recommend, namely, the ſmall forceps, blunt hook, ſciſſars, and curve crotchets, may be had of many inſtrument-makers in *London*.

CON-

CONTENTS.

SECT.

BOOK II.

CHAP. I.

CHAP. II.

SECT.

 bour

CHAP. II.

CHAP.

CHAP. III.

CHAP. IV.

SECT.

CHAP. V.

BOOK IV.

CHAP. I.

NUMB.

CHAP. II.

CHAP. III.

A

INTRODUCTION.

IT muſt be a ſatisfaction to thoſe who begin the ſtudy of any art or ſcience, to be made acquainted with the riſe and progreſs of it; and therefore, I ſhall, by way of introduction, give a ſhort detail of the practice of Midwifery, with the improvements which have been made in it, at different times; as I have been able to collect the circumſtances, from thoſe authors, ancient as well as modern, who have written on the ſubject.

By theſe accounts it ſeems probable, that in the firſt ages, the practice of this art was

alto-

altogether in the hands of women, and that men were never employed but in the utmoſt extremity: indeed it is natural to ſuppoſe, that while the ſimplicity of the early ages remained, women would have recourſe to none but perſons of their own ſex, in diſeaſes peculiar to it; accordingly, we find that in *Egypt* Midwifery was practiſed by women.

In *Athens* a law was made prohibiting women and ſlaves from practiſing phyſick in any ſhape: but the miſtaken modeſty of the ſex rendered it afterwards abſolutely neceſſary to allow free women the privilege of ſharing this art with the men.

In the *Harmonia Gynæciarum*, there are extant ſeveral directions and recipes on the ſubject of Midwifery, collected from the writings of one *Cleopatra*, interſperſed with thoſe of *Moſchion* and *Priſcian*; and ſome people imagine this was no other than the famous *Cleopatra* queen of *Egypt*, becauſe in a preface ſuppoſed to be written by her, ſhe mentions her ſiſter.

Galen

Galen who lived two hundred years after this *Egyptian* queen, adviſes the reader to conſult the writings of one of that name, but does not inform us whether ſhe was or was not that celebrated princeſs; ſo that in all probability, it was ſome other perſon of the ſame name, as the ſtudy and exerciſe of ſuch an art was not at all ſuited to the diſpoſition of ſuch a gay voluptuary as queen *Cleopatra* is deſcribed to have been.

Ætius tranſcribes ſome chapters from the works of one *Aſpaſia*, touching the method of delivering and managing women in natural labours; but gives no account of the place of her reſidence, nor of the time in which ſhe wrote. Several other female practitioners are mentioned by different hiſtorians; but, as none of their writings are extant, and the accounts given of them are moſtly fabulous and foreign to our purpoſe, I ſhall forbear to mention them in this place, and referring the curious to *Le Clerc*'s hiſtory of phyſick, begin with *Hippocrates* the moſt antient writer now extant, upon our ſubject, who may be ſtiled the father of Midwifery as well as medicine; becauſe all the ſucceeding authors, as far down as the latter end of the ſixteenth century, have copied from his works the moſt material things relating to the diſeaſes of women and children, as well as to the obſtetric art. I ſhall therefore give a ſuccinct account of his practice, and in my detail of the other authors, only obſerve the improvements they have made, and the circumſtances in which they have deviated from his method and opinion.

Hippocrates, who practiſed medicine in *Greece*, about 460 years before the chriſtian Æra, no doubt availed himſelf of the obſervations of thoſe who went before him in the exerciſe of the ſame profeſſion. He acquired the higheſt reputation by his wiſe predictions and ſucceſsful practice, and by his uncommon ſagacity and experience greatly improved the healing art.

In his book *de natura Muliebri*, and thoſe *de Mulierum Morbis*, he mentions and deſcribes many diſeaſes peculiar to the female ſex, according to the theory of thoſe times, and preſcribes more medicines for the relief of the ſuffering fair, than are to be met with in all the reſt of his works.

Many of his remedies, indeed, are very ſtrange and uncouth, but a number of them are ſtill accounted excellent in the preſent practice, unleſs his names of them have been miſtaken and miſapplied to other medicines: and although his theory is frequently odd and erroneous, his diagnoſticks, prognoſticks, and method of cure, are often juſt and judicious.

In ſuppreſſions of the Menſes, he firſt of all, orders vomits and purges, then ſharp peſſaries in form of ſuppoſitories, compoſed of lint or wool, with divers kinds of deobſtruent powders, wax and oil, to be introduced into the *Vagina*: he likewiſe preſcribes fumigations, fomentations, and hot baths, together with internal medicines. He obſerves, that ſuch obſtructions produce a pain and ſeeming weight in the lower part of the *Abdomen*, extending to the loins and *Ilia*, attended with a vomiting at intervals, and longings like thoſe of a pregnant woman. If theſe ſymptoms of pain and weight affect the *Hypochondria*, producing ſuffocation and pain in the Head and Neck, the patient is to be relieved by the application of fœtid things to the Noſe, with Caſtor and Flea-bane given internally in wine.

When the menſes flow in too great a quantity, he propoſes a contrary method: he adviſes her to abſtain from bathing and all laxative and diuretic things; orders aſtringent peſſaries for the *Vagina*, and cold applications to the lower parts; preſcribes internally, ſeveral kinds of aſtringent medicines, with the peplium or poppy-ſeed, and cupping glaſſes to be applied to the breaſts. When the violence of the diſcharge is abated, he propoſes purges and vomits, then aſſes milk and a nouriſhing diet, and various kinds of internal and external medicines.

In a *Fluor albus*, he ſays the urine is like that of an aſs; the patient labours under a pain in the lower part of the *Abdomen*, loins

and

and *ilia*, together with a ſwelling in the hands and legs; her eyes water, her complexion becomes wan and yellow, and in walking ſhe is oppreſſed with a difficulty of breathing: In this caſe he preſcribes emeticks and cathарticks, aſſes milk, whey, fomentations, and different kinds of medicines, to deterge and ſtrengthen the genitals.

He mentions many complaints which (in his opinion) proceed from different motions and ſituations of the *Uterus*, and propoſes a good many medicines for the cure. As to his theory of conception, and his opinions about the birth in the ſeventh or eighth month of geſtation, they were actually eſpouſed by all medical writers, till the laſt century.

In his firſt book of the diſeaſes of women, he treats of difficult labours; obſerving, that if a woman is at her full time, ſeized with labour-pains, and cannot, after a long time, be delivered, the child either lies acroſs, or preſents with the feet: for, when the head preſents, the caſe is favourable; whereas if the child lies acroſs, a difficult labour enſues. This aſſertion he illuſtrates by the example of an olive in a narrow mouthed jar, which cannot be ſo eaſily extracted by the middle, as when it preſents with one end. He likewiſe ſays, that the birth will be difficult when the feet preſent, in which caſe, either mother or child, or both (for the moſt part) periſh: Nor is the birth without difficulty when the *Fœtus* is dead, apoplectic or double. He then proceeds to direct us how to relieve the woman of ſeveral complaints to which ſhe may be ſubject after delivery: he deſcribes the method of excluding the *Fœtus*, and of aſſiſting in difficult labours; if the child preſents fair, and is not eaſily delivered, he orders ſternutatories to be adminiſtred, and the patient to ſtop her mouth and noſe, that they may operate the more effectually: She muſt alſo be ſhaken in this manner; let her be faſtened to the bed by a broad band croſſing her breaſt, her legs being bended to the lower part of the bed, the other end of which muſt be ele-

vated

vated by two men, who gently ſhake her by intervals, until her pains expel the child: The parts muſt be anointed with ſome unctuous medicine, and cautiouſly ſeparated; and care muſt be taken, that the *Placenta* immediately follow the child. If the *Fœtus* lies acroſs, preſenting to the *Os uteri*, whether it be alive or dead, he orders it to be puſhed back and turned, ſo as that it may preſent with the head in the natural poſition; and, in order to effect this purpoſe, the woman muſt be laid ſupine on a bed, with her hips raiſed higher than her head. If the child is alive, and preſents with the arm or leg, he adviſes us to return them as ſoon as poſſible, and bring down the head; or if it lies acroſs, preſenting with the ſide or hip, the ſame methods muſt be uſed; then the woman may be refreſhed by ſitting over the ſteams of hot water. The child is to be managed in the ſame manner, when it is dead, and preſents with leg or arm, or both; but if the *Fœtus* cannot be conveniently delivered, on account of the body's being ſwoln, he directs us to bring it away piece-meal, in the following manner: If the head

head presents, let it be opened with a ſmall knife, and the bones of the ſkull being broken, muſt be extracted with a pair of forceps, for fear of hurting the woman; or by an embryulcus, firmly fixed on the Clavicles, it may be extracted by little and little. After the head is delivered in this manner, ſhould the child ſtick at the ſhoulders, he directs us to divide the arms at the articulations; and they being brought away, the reſt of the body, generally, follows with eaſe: but if it will not yet give way, the the whole breaſt muſt be divided; and great care taken that no part of the inteſtines be denudated or wounded, leſt the guts, or their contents, falling out, ſhould retard the operation; then the ribs being broken, and the *Scapulæ* extracted, the reſt of the *Fœtus* will eaſily follow, unleſs the *Abdomen* is ſwoln; in which caſe the belly muſt be punctured, and on the exit of the *Flatus*, the child will be brought along. If part of the child is already delivered, and the reſt will not follow, nor can that which is out be returned, he orders the operator to take away

away as much as he can of it, and pushing up the remainder, turn the head downwards: but, previous to this operation, he advises him to pare his nails, and use a crooked knife; the point and back of which must be covered with the fore finger, at it's introduction, lest it should hurt the *Uterus*.

In his book *de superfœtatione*, he directs us, when the child's head appears without the *Os uteri*, and the rest of the body does not follow, the *Fœtus* being dead, to wet our fingers with water, and introducing them between the *Os uteri* and head, put one into the mouth, and laying hold of it, bring it along. When the body is delivered, and the head remains behind (in those cases when the child comes by the feet) he advises the operator to dip both his hands in water, and introducing them between the *Os uteri* and head of the child, grasp this last with the fingers, and extract it. If the head is in the *Vagina*, it may be delivered in the same manner. When the child remains dead in the *Uterus*, and cannot be de-

delivered, either by the force of nature or medicines, he directs us to introduce the hand, anointed with ſome unctuous cerate, and dividing the parts with an *unguis* fixed on the great finger, bring the *Fœtus* along as before.

In the ſame book of the diſeaſes of women, he gives directions for excluding the *Secundines*, provided they are not expelled in the natural way. He ſays, if the ſecundines come not away immediately after the birth, the woman labours under a pain in her belly and ſide, attended with rigors and a fever, which vaniſh when they are diſcharged; though, for the moſt part, the after-birth putrifies and comes away about the ſixth or ſeventh day, and ſometimes later. In this caſe, he orders the patient to hold her breath, and preſcribes internally, mugwort, cretan dittany, flowers of white violets, leaves of agnus caſtus, with garlick boiled or roaſted, ſmall onions, caſtor, ſpikenard, rue, and black wine.

In

In the book *de Superfœtatione*, after having deſcribed the methods of delivering a dead child, he ſays, if the ſecundines come not away eaſily, the child muſt be left hanging to them, and the woman ſeated on an high ſtool, that the *Fœtus* by its weight may pull them along; and leſt this ſhould be too ſuddenly effected, the child may be laid on wool newly plucked, or on two bladders filled with water, and covered with wool, which being pricked, as the water evacuates, they will ſubſide, and the child ſinking gradually, will gently draw the ſecundines away: but ſhould the navel-ſtring happen to be broke, proper weights muſt be tied to it, in order to anſwer the ſame purpoſe; theſe being the eaſieſt and leaſt hurtful methods of extracting the *Placenta*.

He afterwards obſerves, that if the woman has had a difficult labour, and could not be delivered without the help of machines, the child is generally weak, and therefore the navel-ſtring ought not to be divided, until it ſhall have either urined, ſneezed, or cried aloud; and in the mean

time,

time, it muſt be kept very near the mother: for, though the child does not ſeem to breathe at firſt, nor to give any other ſigns of life, the navel-ſtring by remaining uncut, may be in a little time inflated, and the life of the infant be ſaved.

With regard to the *Lochia* or menſes after delivery, he takes notice, that if they are altogether ſuppreſſed, or the diſcharge inſufficient, and the *Uterus* is indurated, the patient is afflicted with pains in the loins, groins, ſides, thighs and feet, together with an acute fever accompanied with horrors. When the pains happen, unattended with a fever, he orders bathing, and the head to be anointed with oil of dill; and a decoction of mallows with oil of *Cyprus*, to be applied externally, in order to aſſuage the pain. He ſays, in all diſorders where fomentations are neceſſary, the parts ought, afterwards, to be anointed with oil: but, when there is a fever in the caſe, bathing muſt be avoided, warm fomentations uſed, the uterine medicines preſcribed in draughts, and garlick, caſtor or rue boiled with oatmeal: he

likewiſe

likewiſe obſerves, that if the *Uterus* is inflamed after delivery, the patient is in imminent danger of her life, unleſs a ſtool can be procured, or the ſymptom removed by bleeding. He likewiſe aſcribes ſeveral complaints and diſorders of women, to the different poſitions and motions of the *Uterus*, of which laſt, *Plato* who lived immediately after *Hippocrates*, gives a very odd and romantic deſcription, in his *Timæus*. After affirming that there is implanted in the genitals of man, an imperious, headſtrong, inobedient power that endeavours to ſubject every thing to its furious luſts; he ſays, the *Vulva* and *Matrix* of women is alſo an animal ravenous after generation, which being baulked of its deſire for any length of time, is ſo enraged at the diſappointment and delay, that it wanders up and down through the body, obſtructing the circulation, ſtopping the breath, producing ſuffocations and all manner of diſeaſes.

Although we have a piece in *Engliſh*, called *Ariſtotle*'s Midwifery, I find little or nothing of the practice in his works: he hath

hath written on the generation of animals, and we find in him, ſeveral hints curious enough, even upon our ſubject: he tells us, that women ſuffer more than other animals, from uterine geſtation and labour; that thoſe women who take moſt exerciſe, endure both with the greateſt eaſe and ſafety, and that the *Fœtus* in all animals naturally comes by the head, becauſe there being more matter above than below the navel, the head neceſſarily tilts downwards. For this reaſon, he ſays, every birth in which the head preſents, is natural, and thoſe unnatural in which the feet, or any other part of the body, come foremoſt.

We have nothing written on the ſubject of Midwifery, from his time, to that of *Celſus*, who is ſuppoſed to have lived in the reign of the emperor *Tiberius*. This author hath given a chapter on the delivery of dead children, and the *Placenta*, in which he hath copied from *Hippocrates*, though he is more full than his maſter, and mentions ſeveral improvements on his practice. After having given directions with regard to the woman's poſition, he adviſes the operator

to

to introduce one finger after another until the whole hand ſhall gain admittance: he ſays that the largeneſs of the *Uterus*, and the ſtrength and courage of the patient, are great advantages to the birth; that the woman's *Abdomen* and extremities muſt be kept as warm as poſſible; that we muſt not wait until an inflammation is produced, but aſſiſt her without delay; becauſe ſhould her body be ſwelled, we can neither introduce our hands, nor deliver the child, without great difficulty; and vomittings, tremors, and convulſions often enſue. When the crotchet is fixed upon the Head, he directs us to pull with caution, leſt the inſtrument ſhould give way, and lacerate the mouth of the womb; by which means the woman would be thrown into convulſions and imminent danger of her life. When the feet preſent, he ſays the child is eaſily delivered, by laying hold on them, with the hands, and ſo bringing them along. If the *Fœtus* lies acroſs, and cannot be brought down, he orders the crotchet to be fixed on the armpit, and drawn along by little and little: by theſe endeavours the neck will be almoſt doubled, and the head bent backwards; in which caſe, this laſt muſt be ſeparated from the body, and the whole extracted piece-meal. The operation (he ſays) muſt be performed with a crotchet, the internal ſurface of which is edged, and the head be brought away before the body; becauſe, if the greateſt part be extracted firſt, and the head left alone in the *Uterus*, the caſe will be attended with great difficulty and danger. Neverthelesſ, ſhould this misfortune happen, he directs a double cloth to be laid on the woman's belly, and a ſkilful aſſiſtant to ſtand at her left ſide, and with both hands on the *Abdomen*, to preſs from ſide to ſide, with a view of forcing the head againſt the *Os Uteri*; which being effected, it muſt be delivered by fixing the crotchet in the ſkull. With regard to the *Placenta*, he directs us to deliver it in this manner: The child being delivered, muſt be given to a ſervant, who holds it on the palms of his hands, while the operator gently pulls the umbilical cord, for fear of breaking it, and tracing it with his right hand as far as the *Secundines*, ſeparates the *Placenta* from the *Uterus* with his fingers, and extracts it intire, together with the gru-

mous

mous blood: then the woman's thighs being placed cloſe together, ſhe muſt be kept in a moderately warm room, free from wind, and a cloth dipped in *Oxyrrhodon* muſt be laid on her *Abdomen*: the reſt of the cure conſiſting in the application of thoſe things which are uſed in inflammations and wounds of the tendons.

Moſchion, who is ſuppoſed to have lived at *Rome* in the reign of *Nero*, ſays, That in difficult births, the parts are firſt of all to be relaxed with oil: if the paſſage of the urine is obſtructed by a ſtone in the neck of the bladder, he adviſes us to draw off the water with a catheter; if the *Fæces* are indurated, he preſcribes a clyſter, and orders the membranes to be pierced with a lancet. He ſays, the beſt poſition is that of the head preſenting, the hands and feet being mingled and diſpoſed along the ſides. If the poſition is not right, and cannot be amended by putting the woman in proper poſtures, he adviſes us to introduce the hand, when the *Os Uteri* is opened, and turn the child. If a foot preſents (ſays he) puſh it back, and bring the *Fœtus* by both feet, the arms being preſſed down along the ſides: if the knee or hip preſents, they muſt be alſo puſhed back, and the child brought by the feet: if the back preſents, introduce the hand, and alter the poſition, by turning to the feet, or to the head, if it be neareſt; and if the head is large, it muſt be opened, *&c.*

Rufus Epheſius, who lived in the reign of *Trajan*, gives a ſhort account of the *Uterus* and its appendages, and deſcribes thoſe tubes which are now called Fallopian, as opening into the cavity of the womb; though *Galen* arrogates this diſcovery to himſelf, ſo particularly, as to ſay upon this ſubject, that he was ſurprized to find they had eſcaped the notice of the common herd of anatomiſts; but more eſpecially amazed that a man of *Herophilus*'s accuracy, ſhould be ignorant of them: and *Rufus* has expreſly mentioned the opinion of *Herophilus*, on this particular.

Galen was born in the time of the emperor *Adrian*, *Anno Dom.* 131. about ſix hundred years after *Hippocrates*, upon whoſe works he writes commentaries, and gives ſome

ſome reaſonable aphoriſms relating to women and children: we have two books of his writing, *de Semine*; (the third being accounted ſpurious) one, *de Uteri Diſſectione*, *de Fœtuum Formatione*, *de Septimenſtri Partu*, *Lib.* 14 & 15. *de uſu Partium.* He hath alſo written ſeveral books on anatomy and phyſiology, but nothing *de Morbis Mulierum.* In his phyſiology he is prolix and inaccurate: his anatomy is pretty exact in many things; but, upon the whole, he contains little or nothing to our purpoſe.

In *Oribaſius*, who was phyſician to *Julian*, we have a deſcription of the parts, and in ſeveral places of his works, an account of the medicines uſed by the antients in the diſeaſes of women and children: he has alſo a chapter on the choice of a nurſe, and another upon the milk, but ſays nothing of the operation.

Ætius, who (according to *Le Clerc*) lived in the end of the fourth, but in the opinion of Dr. *Friend*, in the end of the fifth century, was likewiſe a collector from the antients: for neither he nor *Oribaſius* can be

 ſtiled

ſtiled original writers: the laſt indeed, copied from none (almoſt) but *Galen*; whereas the other compiled from all the authors that went before him, many of whom would have been loſt in oblivion, had not they been mentioned in his works; he was ſtiled *Simia Galeni*, or *Galen*'s ape: he is very particular upon the diſeaſes and management of women; his fourth *Sermo* of the 4th *Tetrab* being expreſly written on this ſubject, and containing almoſt every thing which had been ſaid before him.

In his firſt chapter, *De uteri ſitu, magnitudine ac forma*, he diſtinctly divides the womb into a fundus and neck, and deſcribes the *Os Tincæ*, as ending in the *Sinus Muliebris, ſive Pudendum*, which plainly appears to be no other than what we now call the *Vagina*; for, he ſays, it is above ſix inches in length; but his deſcription of the figure of the *Uterus* is imperfect. His ſeventh chapter treats of conception, from *Soranus*. The tenth of the *Pica*, taken from ſome of *Galen*'s works that are loſt. His deſcription of this diſeaſe, is to the following purpoſe. Young women with child have vitiated

ated appetites, and long for earth, aſhes, coal, ſhells, &c. The diſtemper continues till the ſecond or third month of geſtation; but commonly abates in the fourth. To remedy the nauſea and vomiting that attend it, he orders aloes, dried mint, and other ſtomachics.

In his twelfth and fifteenth chapters, he gives a detail of *Aſpaſia*'s practice in the care and management of women, during pregnancy, and in time of labour; but the greateſt part of theſe and the other chapters, are taken from *Hippocrates*, to whom he has made a few inſignificant additions, until we come to the twentieth and ſecond, in which there is a very full and diſtinct account of difficult births.

Among the cauſes that produce difficult labours, he enumerates weakneſs of mind or body, or both, a confined *Uterus*, a narrow paſſage, natural ſmallneſs of the parts, obliquity of the neck of the *Uterus*, a fleſhy ſubſtance adhering to the *Cervix* or mouth of the womb, inflammation, abſceſs or induration of the parts, rigidity of the membranes, premature diſcharge of the waters, which ought to be detained for moiſtening and lubricating the parts, a ſtone preſſing againſt the neck of the bladder, and extraordinary fatneſs; an *Anchyloſis* of the *Oſſa Pubis* at their juncture, by which they are hindered from ſeparating in time of parturition, too great preſſure of the *Uterus* on the cavity of the loins, or too great quantity of *Fœces* and urine retained in the *Rectum* and bladder, an enfeebled conſtitution, advanced age, ſlender make, and greenneſs of years attended with weakneſs and inexperience.

He obſerves, that difficult labours likewiſe proceed from circumſtances belonging to the child that is to be born: from the extraordinary ſize of the body, or any part of it; from its being unable (through weakneſs) to facilitate the birth by its leaping and motion: from the crowding of two or three *Fœtuſes*: from twins preſenting together at the mouth of the womb: from the death of the child, as it can give no

aſ-

aſſiſtance in promoting labour: from its tumefaction after death, and wrong preſentation.

He ſays, the natural poſition is when the head preſents and comes forwards, the hands being extended along the thighs; and the preternatural, that in which the head is turned either to the right or left ſide of the *Uterus*; when one or both hands preſent, and the legs within are ſeparated from one another: that the danger is not great when the feet preſent, eſpecially if the child comes forwards with the hands along the thighs; and that if, while one leg preſents, the other is kept up or bent in the *Vagina*, this laſt muſt be brought down: nor is the difficulty great in thoſe that lie acroſs, a circumſtance that may happen in three different ways; namely, when the child preſents with either ſide, or with the belly: Neverthelefs, he obſerves, that the caſe is eaſieſt when the ſide preſents, becauſe there is more room for the operator to introduce his hand, and turn the *Fœtus* ſo as that it may come either by the

the head or feet. The worſt poſition, he ſays, is when the child preſents double, eſpecially if the hip-bones come foremoſt: This double preſentation happens with the hips, the head and legs, and the belly; in which laſt caſe, he obſerves, that if the *Abdomen* is opened, and the intrails taken out, the parts collapſe, and the poſition is eaſily altered.

Over and above the fore-mentioned cauſes of difficult labour, he affirms, it may be owing to an over thickneſs or thinneſs of the membranes, which break too late or too ſoon; as alſo to external cauſes, ſuch as cold weather, by which the pores and paſſages of the body are conſtringed; or very hot weather, by which they are too much relaxed. All theſe circumſtances (he ſays) ought to be minutely enquired into, and duly conſidered, by the phyſician who directs the midwife; nor ought this laſt to be permitted to tear or ſtretch the parts with violence. If the difficulty proceeds from the form of the *Pelvis*, he directs the woman to be ſeated on a ſtool, her knees being bent

and

and kept aſunder; by which means the *Vulva* will be dilated, and the *Cervix* extended in a ſtreight line: And thoſe that are groſs or fat, are to be placed in the ſame manner. If the difficulty ariſes from ſtraitneſs, ſtupor or contractions, he ſays, it will be proper to relax the parts, by ſeating the patient over warm ſteams and fumigations, in a place conveniently warmed; by pour-into the *Vagina* warmed oils, and by the application of emollient ointments and cataplaſms: For this purpoſe, he likewiſe recommends the warm bath (unleſs a fever or other complaint render it improper). Some, he obſerves, are carried about in a litter, in a warm place; and others have been ſubjected to violent concuſſions: but thoſe who, by a weak, looſe habit, are too much enfeebled to undergo labour, ought to be treated with preſcriptions that conſolidate, ſtrengthen, and conſtringe: They ought to be ſprinkled with perfumes and vinegar, anointed with cooling ointments of wine and oil of roſes, and ſit over infuſions of roſes, myrtle, pomegranates, and vine twigs.

If

If the difficulty is owing to the præternatural poſition of the *Fœtus*, it muſt be as much as poſſible reduced into the natural way. If the foot or hand is protruded, the child muſt not be pulled by either; the limb muſt be returned, twiſted, or lopt off, and the ſhoulder or hip moved with the fingers into a more convenient ſituation. When the whole body of the *Fœtus* is ſtrongly preſſed down in a wrong poſition, he adviſes us to raiſe it to the uppermoſt part of the *Uterus*, and turn it downwards again in a right poſture: This operation muſt be performed gently and ſlowly, without violence; oil being frequently injected into the parts, that no injury may be ſuſtained by either mother or child. If the mouth of the womb continues cloſe ſhut, it muſt be ſoftned and relaxed by oily medicines: If there is a ſtone in the neck of the bladder, it muſt be puſhed up with the catheter, and the urine (if in great quantity) drawn off. If the *Rectum* is filled with *Fæces*, it muſt be evacuated by clyſters: And proper methods are

are to be taken, when delivery is prevented by inflammation, abſceſs, ulcer, ſoft or hard tumors, or any other ſuch obſtacles.

If the difficulty proceeds from a fleſhy ſubſtance adhering to the neck of the womb, or from a thick membrane found in thoſe women who are imperforated, the obſtacle in both caſes muſt be removed by the knife; and if the membranes that ſurround the child are too rigid to give way at the proper time, they muſt be cut without delay: If, on the contrary, the waters are diſcharged too ſoon, ſo as that the parts are left dry, the want of them muſt be ſupplied with lubricating injections, made with the whites of eggs, decoctions of mallows, fenugrec and the cream of barley ptiſan.

If the difficulty proceeds from the ſmallneſs or ſtrong contraction of the *Uterus*, the parts are likewiſe to be rendered ſoft and diſtenſile with lubricating ointments and fomentations; the mouth of the womb muſt be dilated with the fingers, and the child

ex-

extracted by force; but should this method fail, the *Fœtus* must be cut in pieces, and brought away by little and little. This (he says) is the only resource when the *Fœtus* is too large, and the most proper when it is dead; and its death may be certainly pronounced, when the presenting part is felt cold and without motion. When two or three children present in the neck of the *Uterus*, those that are highest must be raised up to the *Fundus*, until the lowest be first delivered.

If the difficulty is owing to the excessive largeness of the head, breast, or belly, he says, it will be absolutely necessary to open these cavities; and observes, that the most proper time for placing the woman in labour upon the stool, is when the membranes are felt presenting in a round extended bag.

His twentieth and third chapter contains the method of extraction and exsection of the *Fœtus*, from *Philomenus*; and is an accurate detail of the operations recommended above.

above. He ſays, before the operator begins to deliver by exſection, he ought to conſider the ſtrength of the patient, and determine with himſelf, whether or not there is a probability of ſaving her life; becauſe, if ſhe is exhauſted, enervated, lethargic, ſeized with convulſions, *ſubſultus tendinum*, with a diſordered pulſe, it is better to decline the operation, than run the riſque of her periſhing under his hands: But if he thinks her ſtrength and courage ſufficient for the occaſion, let her be laid in bed, on her back, her head being low, and her legs held aſunder by ſtrong experienced women; ſhe may take by way of cordial, two or three mouthfuls of bread dipped in wine, in order to prevent her fainting; for which purpoſe, her face may be alſo ſprinkled with wine during the operation. The chirurgeon having opened the *Pudenda* with an inſtrument, and obſerved the ſource of the difficulty, whether tumor, callus, or any of the cauſes already mentioned, he muſt take hold of it with a forceps, and amputate with a biſtory: If a membrane obſtructs the mouth of the womb,

womb, it muſt be divided: If the delivery is prevented by the rigidity of the membranes that invelop the *Fœtus*, they muſt be pinched up with a pair of ſmall forceps, and cut with a ſharp knife; then the perforation may be dilated with the fingers, ſo as to effect a ſufficient opening for the paſſage of the child.

If the paſſage is obſtructed by the head of the *Fœtus*, it muſt be turned and delivered by the feet; but if the head is ſo impacted, as that it cannot poſſibly be returned, a hook or crochet muſt be fixed in the eye, mouth, or over the chin, and in this manner the child may be extracted with the operator's right hand: but, beſides this crochet, which ought to be gently introduced, and guarded with the fingers of the left hand, another muſt be inſinuated in the ſame manner, and fixed on the oppoſite ſide, that the head may be extracted more equally, without ſticking in one place, and one of the inſtruments hold, in caſe the other ſhould ſlip; and when theſe crochets are properly applied, the operator muſt pull, not only in a ſtreight line, but alſo from ſide to ſide.

He directs us to introduce our fingers beſmeared with unctuous medicines, betwixt the mouth of the womb and the impacted body, in order to lubricate it all round. When the *Fœtus* is delivered as far as the middle, the extracting inſtrument muſt be fixed in the upper parts: if the head is either naturally too large or dropſical, it muſt be opened with a ſharp-pointed knife, that it may be evacuated, contracted, and delivered: But if, notwithſtanding this operation, it cannot be brought along, the ſkull muſt be ſqueezed together, the bones pulled out with the fingers or bone-forceps, and the crochet fixed for delivery. But if, after the head is extracted, there ſhould be a contraction round the thorax, a perforation muſt be made near the clavicles, into the cavity of the breaſt, that the bulk may be diminiſhed by the evacuation of the contained humours: If the child is dead, and the belly diſtended with air or water, the

Abdomen muſt alſo be opened, and, if need be, the inteſtines extracted.

If the arm preſents, it muſt be ſeparated at the joint of the ſhoulder: For this purpoſe, a cloth muſt be wrapt round it, that it may not ſlip while it is pulled down to the ſhoulder; then opening the *Labia*, the joint will appear at which the limb may be taken off: This amputation being performed, the head muſt be puſhed up, and the *Fœtus* delivered. The ſame method muſt be purſued when both arms preſent, and when, though the feet are forced out, the reſt of the body will not follow; in which caſe, the legs muſt be ſeparated at the groins.

If, when the *Fœtus* preſents double, and cannot be raiſed up, the head is fartheſt down, the bones of the ſkull are to be ſqueezed together, without opening the ſcalp or ſkin, and the crochet being fixed in ſome part of it, will bring it forth, the body following in a ſtreight line: but if he legs are neareſt, they muſt be amputated at at the *Coxa*, and the hips puſhed up, ſo as to allow the head to be ſqueezed and prepared for extraction. When the *Fœtus* preſents double, he ſays, it is better to divide the head from the body, than to puſh up the *Thorax*, and deliver by the feet: But ſhould the reſt of the body be delivered, and the head left behind, the left hand anointed muſt be introduced into the *Uterus*, and the head being brought down with the fingers to the mouth of the womb, one or two crochets muſt be fixed on it, in order to bring it along; the moſt proper places in the head for the application of this inſtrument, being the eyes, ears, mouth, or under the chin: For the extraction of the *Thorax*, it may be fixed in the armpits, clavicles, *Præcordia*, breaſt, and joints of the back and neck: For the lower parts, on the *Pubis*, or in the *Pudenda* of female children.

If the mouth of the womb be ſhut by an inflammation, he cautions us againſt uſing any violence; but orders it to be ſoftened and relaxed by oily medicines, fumigations, baths, cataplaſms; by theſe means the inflammation will be leſſened or removed, and the *Os internum* dilated ſo as to allow the *Fœtus* to be delivered. If the body hath been extracted piece-meal, he directs the parts to be laid together, in order to obſerve if the whole is delivered, and if any thing remains, it muſt be extracted without delay.

In his twentieth and fourth chapter, (the ſubſtance of which is alſo taken from *Philumenus*) he lays down the following directions for extracting the ſecundines.

The *Os internum* (when the ſecundines are detained) is ſometimes ſhut, ſometimes open, and often inflamed; the *Placenta* ſometimes adhering to the *Fundus*, and ſometimes in a ſtate of ſeparation. If the *Os internum* is open, and the ſecundines, ſeparated from the *Uterus*, lie rolled up like a ball, they are eaſily extracted by introducing the left hand warmed and anointed; and after

5 having

having taken hold of them, drawing them gently down from ſide to ſide, and not ſtreight forwards, for fear of a *Prolapſus vulvæ*. If the *Os uteri* is ſhut, it muſt be opened ſlowly with the finger, after it hath been lubricated with oil or auxunge: If this method ſhould fail, a pultice of barley-meal malaxed with oil, muſt be applied to the belly, the oily injections repeated; and if the patient's ſtrength will permit, ſhe muſt take ſternutatories of caſtor and pepper, and potions of thoſe medicines that bring down the *Menſes*, ſitting at the ſame over a fumigation.

All theſe things muſt be tried on the firſt and ſecond days, and if they ſucceed, ſo as to open the mouth of the womb, the ſecundines will be eaſily extracted as above: but, if all theſe methods fail, the woman muſt be no longer fatigued; they will in a few days putrify and come off in a diſſolved ſanies; and ſhould the fœtid ſmell affect the head and ſtomach, he preſcribes ſuch medicines as are uſed in obſtructions of the *Menſes.*

His next chapter, which is taken from *Aſpaſia*, treats of the management of women after delivery; and he writes ſeveral more on the diſeaſes incident to women, ſuch as inflammations, impoſtumes, and cancers of the breaſt and *uterus*; compiled from *Philomenus*, *Leonides*, *Archigenus*, *Philagrius*, *Soranus*, *Rufus*, *Aſpaſia*, and *Aſclepiades.*

The next conſiderable author on this ſubject, is *Paulus Ægineta*, whom *Le Clerc* ſuppoſes to have lived in the latter end of the fourth century; though Dr. *Friend* brings him down to the ſeventh. He was the laſt of the old *Greek* medical writers, and the firſt inſtance on record, of a profeſs'd man-midwife: for ſo he was called by the *Arabians*, and accordingly begins his book with diſorders incident to pregnant women.

His method of practice is much the ſame with that of *Ætius* and *Philomenus*, as above deſcribed; and though not ſo full as they, he is very diſtinct and particular. He tells us in his preface, that he had collected from others; and although he was the firſt who had the name of man-midwife from the *Arabians*, the writings of *Ætius* plainly ſhew, that there had been many male-practioners before him. In the ſeventy-ſixth chapter of his third book, which treats of difficult births, he gives the appellation of natural to all thoſe in which the head or feet preſent; and all other poſitions he deems præternatural.

In another place, he obſerves, that the woman ought to be ſeated on the ſtool or chair, when, by the touch, the mouth of the womb is felt open, and the membranes puſhed down. As to his method of extracting a dead child and the *Placenta*, it is much the ſame with that already deſcribed from *Philumenus*, in the preceding article.

Paulus is ſuppoſed to have ſtudied at *Alexandria*: for, long before his time, the *Roman* empire in the weſt had been overrun and ruined by the *Goths* and *Vandals*.

Soon after this period, learning began to decline in the eaſt; the ſchools of *Alexandria* were removed to *Antioch* and *Haran* by the *Saracens*, who ſubdued *Egypt*, and deſtroyed the *Roman* empire in *Aſia*, and then the *Greek* phyſicians were tranſlated into the *Syriac* and *Arabic*: at leaſt, the *Arabians* copied from them. This ſubject is fully diſcuſſed by Dr. *Friend*, in his hiſtory of phyſick.

Serapian, one of the firſt *Arabian* writers, in his *Tractatus Quintus* has ſeveral chapters on the diſeaſes of pregnant women, with the method of cure.

The next author of any note, belonging to this country, was *Rhazes*; who, in the latter end of the ninth century, lived at *Bagdat*. Like other ſyſtematic writers in phyſick, he hath treated of the diſeaſes of women; and written one book expreſly on the diſeaſes of children.

In the laſt chapter of his *Liber Diviſionum*, he orders the membranes, when they are too tough, to be pierced with the nail of of the finger, or with a little knife: And if the waters are diſcharged a long time before delivery, ſo that the parts remain dry, he directs us to anoint them with oily cerates.

Avicenna lived at *Iſpahan* about the year one thouſand, and was ſo famous for his writings all over *Aſia* and *Europe*, that no other doctrine was taught in the ſchools of phyſick, till the reſtoration of learning. He is a voluminous author, treats largely of every part of midwifery, ſo far as it was known in his time; copying from thoſe that went before him: the operation for the dead child he takes from *Paulus*; the extraction of the ſecundines from *Philumenus*; and the uſe of the fillet from his countryman *Rhazes*. He is very full on all the diſeaſes of women, relating to the *Menſes*, uterine geſtation, and delivery.

In all præternatural caſes, he ſays, the head ought to be reduced into the natural poſition; but ſhould this be found impracticable, he adviſes us to deliver by the feet.

He

He alledges, that the head is the only natural way of preſenting, and that all other poſitions are præternatural; though of theſe, the eaſieſt is when the *Fœtus* preſents with the feet.

He recommends all the old methods for aſſiſting in natural labours, and if the woman cannot be delivered by theſe, he orders a fillet to be fixed over the head: If that cannot be done, to extract with the forceps; and ſhould theſe fail, to open the ſkull; by which means, the contents will be evacuated, the head diminiſhed, and the *Fœtus* eaſily delivered.

The next *Arabian* medical writer is *Albucaſis*, who, in the eleventh or twelfth century, lived at *Cyropolis*, a city of *Media*, on the *Caſpian* Sea; and it appears from an *Arabian* manuſcript, in the *Bodleian* library, that this is the ſame perſon who was alſo known by the name of *Alſaharavius*.

He hath written on natural labours in the ſame way with his predeceſſors, adviſing us

to

to aſſiſt the birth with fomentations, and ointments, and by reducing the child into the natural poſition, when any other part than the head preſents. His operation for extracting the dead child, is literally the ſame with that deſcribed by *Ætius*; but whether he copied it from that author, or from other *Arabians* his predeceſſors, is uncertain.

What is moſt particular in this author is, the deſcription and figures of the inſtruments then uſed in midwifery; namely, a vertigo for opening the matrix, which ſeems to be much of the ſame contrivance with that which *Rhazes* calls the *Torculum volvens*. He likewiſe exhibits the figures of two other inſtruments for the ſame purpoſe; but not one of the three in the leaſt reſembles the *Speculum matricis*, deſcribed in later writers. An *Impellens*, to keep up the body of the child while the operator endeavours to reduce the head into the natural poſition. Two kinds of forceps, of a circular form, furniſhed with teeth on the inſide, to ſqueeze and cruſh the head, when it

is

is of an extraordinary bigneſs; the larger he calls *Almiſdach*, the other *Miſdach*: And two different kinds of crochets.

After the twelfth century, phyſick began to decline in *Aſia*. *Theodore Gaza* brought the *Greek* manuſcripts from *Conſtantinople*, after that city was taken in the year 1453; and about this time, the art of printing being found out, all the knowledge of the ancients was ſoon diſperſed over *Europe*.

In the next century, the practice of phyſick began to be encouraged in *England*. *Linacre*, born at *Canterbury*, and choſen Fellow of *All-ſouls*, in *Oxford*, in the year 1484, was a man of learning, and projected the foundation of the college of phyſicians in *London*; for which he obtained a patent from King *Henry* VIII. and was himſelf preſident of it till the day of his death.

In the year 1565, one Dr. *Raynalde* publiſhed a book on midwifery, which he had tranſlated into *Engliſh* from the original *Latin*.

Latin. He informs the reader in his proluge (as he terms it) that the book, which was called *De partu hominis*, had been tranſlated about two or three years before, at the requeſt of ſome women, by a ſtudious and diligent clark; who having performed the taſk incorrectly, he (Dr. *Raynalde*) had been at great pains to reviſe and enlarge it in another tranſlation: He alſo obſerves, that the *Latin* edition had been formerly publiſhed in *Dutch*, *French*, *Spaniſh*, and other languages *.

The author of this performance (contrary to the opinions of all other writers) ſays, when the child preſents in the natural way with the head, that the face and foreparts of the *Fœtus* are towards the foreparts of the mother; and that if any other part preſents, the poſition is preternatural. He obſerves, that in *France* and *Germany*, the woman is commonly placed in a ſitting poſition,

* This author was *Eucharius Rhodion*, whoſe book was in great eſteem all over *Germany*; and in the year 1532, being tranſlated into *Latin* and other languages, from the original *High Dutch*, became univerſally the woman's book over all *Europe*, and was introduced into *England*; where it was tranſlated by this Dr. *Raynalde*, who, nevertheleſs, has taken great liberties with his author.

on

on a ſtool made in form of a compaſs; and adviſes us, in all preternatural caſes, to turn the child to the natural poſition, even when the feet preſent: But if this ſhould be impracticable, to bring it footling, and, in extracting, to bind the feet together with a linen cloth. This, however, he pronounces a very jeopardous labour. He directs us to provoke and promote the delivery with fumigations and peſſaries, and to preſcribe internally, aſſa-fœtida, myrrh, caſtor, and ſtorax: From which circumſtances, he ſeems to have copied from the ancient writers.

Several authors of note lived and wrote in the ſixteenth century, or betwixt the years 1530 and 1590, upon the diſeaſes of pregnant women, and the different methods of delivery. A collection of the moſt remarkable among theſe writers, who are called the old moderns, was publiſhed at *Baſil* 1586, in a large quarto, intitled *Gynæciorum*; and afterwards, in 1597, republiſhed at *Straſburg* in folio, by *Iſrael Spachius*, profeſſor of medicine in that city, with the addition of two authors, who had not been men-

mentioned in the firſt. At the head of this collection, is *Felix Platerus*, born at *Baſil:* He publiſhed tables, explaining the uſe and ſtructure of the parts of generation proper to women.

The next is an edition of *Moſchion* (already mentioned) reviſed and corrected by *Conradus Geſnerus*, and publiſhed by his ſcholar *Caſparus Wolphius Tigurinus*.

The third is the *Harmonia Gynæciorum* of *Cleopatra*, *Moſchion*, *Theodorus Priſcianus*, and other uncertain authors, publiſhed together in one piece, and freed from repetitions and ſuperfluities, by the ſame *Caſparus Wolphius*.

Then follows *Eros* or *Trotula*, publiſhed among the old *Latin* writers at *Venice*, by the ſons of *Aldus*.

The fifth place is held by *Nicholaus Rochæus*, a *Frenchman*, whoſe works, publiſhed at *Paris*, are taken from the *Greeks* and *Arabians*; though he hath added ſome obſervations of his own. In his twentieth and

eighth

eighth chapter, he ſays, if the child is large, the *Os uteri* muſt be dilated; if the hand or foot preſents, neither muſt be laid hold on; but the operator, introducing his hand to the buttock or ſhoulder, muſt reduce the *Fœtus* into the natural ſituation, that is, when it preſents with the head. His thirtieth chapter contains directions for extracting the *Placenta* when it adheres: The *Os uteri* muſt be dilated, and the accoucheur taking hold of the *Funis*, muſt pull gently from ſide to ſide, leſt the *Uterus* ſhould be brought down; then more ſtrength muſt be exerted by degrees, until the ſecundines are brought away. His thirty-ſecond chapter treats of monſters.

Ludovicus Bonaciolus of *Ferrara*, is the ſixth: His works were publiſhed at *Straſbourg*.

The ſeventh is *Jacobus Silvius* of *Amiens*, in *Picardy*.

Then comes *Jacobus Ruffus*, who publiſhed at *Zurich*, in *Switzerland*, and at *Franckfort*. He is the firſt that gives a draught

draught of the *Speculum matricis*, for dilating the *Os internum*, which he directs to be ſtretched in width; but by no means lengthways, leſt, the ligaments breaking, the womb ſhould fall down. When the feet preſent, and the hands are ſtretched along the ſides, he adviſes us to deliver footling; but if the hands are up over the head, he ſays the child ought not to be brought by the feet, unleſs the head be very ſmall. If the knees preſent, he orders them to be puſhed up, and the child to be delivered by the feet: but if the breech comes firſt, it muſt be reduced, and the *Fœtus* brought by the head. The ſame practice he recommends in the preſentation of the hands, ſhoulder, or hands and feet together.

He is ſucceeded by *Hieron Mercurialis*, who lived at *Padua*, *Venice*, and *Bologna*, and practiſed much in the ſame manner.

The tenth is *Johannes Baptiſta Montanus* of *Padua*.

Victor Trincavillus, of *Venice*, is the next.

Albertus Battonus, of *Padua*, is the twelfth.

After him comes *Joannes le Bon Heteropolitanus*.

The author, who holds the next place in this collection, is *Ambrosius Paræus*, the famous restorer and improver of Midwifery: He lived at *Paris*, and his works were translated into *Latin* by *Jacob Guillemeau*.

Next to him *Spachius* places *Albucasis*, the *Arabian*, already mentioned. Then

Franciscus Roussètus, who wrote on the *Cæsarian* operation: His work was translated from *French* by *Casparus Bauhinus*; and several of his cases are published in the memoirs of the academy of surgeons, by *M. Simon*.

The seventeenth is *Lithopedus Senonensis*.

Casparus Bauhinus, professor at *Basil*, is the eighteenth.

Then

Then *Mauriceus Cordæus*, of *Rheims* and *Paris*.

The twentieth is *Martinus Akakia*, of *Paris*; and the laſt is *Ludovicus Mercatus*, a *Spaniard*.----This author ſays, if the child does not preſent with the head or feet, the caſe is dangerous, and præternatural; nor is the preſentation of the feet without hazard and difficulty. In laborious labours, if the woman be young and vigorous, he preſcribes bleeding in the foot, after *Hippocrates*; but is againſt the uſe of the bath.

If the *Fœtus* comes double, or preſents wrong, he directs us to puſh it up, and bring down the head, if poſſible; which ought alſo to be our aim, when the hand or foot preſents. He orders the fingers to be introduced as *Paulus* directs, (*digitis in unum conductis*) that is, the fingers and thumb formed into the ſhape of a cone. He exclaims againſt the *Cæſarian* operation as an unchriſtian undertaking; directs us, when the *Placenta* adheres, to introduce the hand,

and pull the *Funis* gently from ſide to ſide; and recommends ſneezing to the woman, as conducive to its expulſion,

When he treats of the manner of extracting a dead child, he ſays, with *Ætius*, we ought firſt to conſider whether or not the woman has ſtrength ſufficient to bear the operation; then gives the method of *Hippocrates*, and in the next page deſcribes the manner of *Ætius*.

Having thus given a ſhort ſketch of the authors collected by *Spachius*, I ſhall return to *Paræus*, who (as I have already hinted) was the firſt modern that made any conſiderable improvements in Midwifery; which continued, to his time without any material alteration, even after the other branches of phyſick had been improved. For example, if the child did not preſent in the natural way, they ſhook and altered the poſition of the woman, by which means they imagined the *Fœtus* would turn to the right poſture; or they attempted to move it ſo as that it ſhould preſent with the head: If this could not

not be effected, and the feet were near at hand, they brought it footling; but if they failed in this attempt, the child was supposed to be dead, and extracted with crochets and hooks of various kinds; and if it could not be delivered in that manner, on account of its extraordinary size, or the narrowness of the *Pelvis*, they dismembered and separated the body with crooked and streight knives, and then extracted it piecemeal.

Paræus was the first that deviated from this practice, and expressly orders the child to be turned and brought away by the feet in all præternatural cases. He says, the most natural case is that in which the child presents with the head, and is delivered immediately on the discharge of the waters: it is more difficult when the *Fœtus* comes by the feet, and still more so, in the presentation of the arm and legs together, the back, belly, arm alone, or any other unnatural position. He directs us to bring away the secundines immediately after the child is delivered: He retains the old notions relating to the diseases and medicines; for the antient theory was not alter'd till after the great *Harvey* found out the circulation of the blood.

Cotemporary with him, was *Jacobus Ruef*, who practiſed at *Franckfort*, and in his writings recommends the method of the antients: A circumſtance from which we learn, that the improvements had not then reached *Germany*. Indeed they were very much retarded by the falſe modeſty of the women, who were ſhy of male practitioners; and by the miſtaken notions which were at that time entertained of the ſtructure of the *Uterus*; for all the deſcriptions, till the time of *Veſalius*, were very imperfect; and the womb in women ſuppoſed to be formed of different cells, reſembling that of the brute ſpecies.

Jacobus Guillemeau was the pupil of *Ambroſius Paræus*, adopted and confirmed his maſter's practice, and has written with learning and judgment.

About the end of the ſixteenth century, or in *Paræus'* time, ſurgery in general was

more

more cultivated and improved in *Paris* than in any other part of the world, by means of the hoſpitals which had been from time to time erected, eſpecially the *Hotel Dieu*, into which poor women with child, deſtitute of the neceſſaries of life, were admitted.

By ſuch opportunities, the ſurgeons improved their knowledge in Midwifery; and, by degrees, eſtabliſhed a better method of practice: The ſucceſs that attended which, together with the progreſs of polite literature that began to flouriſh about this time in *France*, got the better of thoſe ridiculous prejudices which the fair ſex had been uſed to entertain, and they had recourſe to the aſſiſtance of men in all difficult caſes of Midwifery. This conduct was juſtified by experience; and the lives of many women and children were ſaved by the ſkill of the man-practitioner.

In the year 1668, *Francis Mauriceau*, after an extenſive practice for ſeveral years, in the *Hotel Dieu* and city of *Paris*, publiſhed a treatiſe on Midwifery, which exceeded every thing before made public on that ſubject. He deſcribes the bones of the *Pelvis*, and all the parts ſubſervient to generation; the diſeaſes incident to pregnant women, with the methods of prevention and cure; and, after having given a full and diſtinct account of all the different labours, and the way of delivering in each caſe, concludes his work with the diſeaſes of women and children.

His method of practice was nearly the ſame with that of *Paræus* and *Guillemeau*; but he is much fuller than either. In laborious caſes, when the head preſents, and cannot be delivered by the labour-pains, he orders a fillet, or ſtripe of linen, to be ſlit in the middle, and ſlipped over the head: This contrivance hath ſince been improved with laces, by which it is contracted on the head. It is introduced by three different inſtruments, fixed with a great deal of trouble, and, after all, of very little uſe.

He alſo invented a tire-tête, which cannot be applied until the ſkull is opened with a knife;

knife; consequently can be of no service in saving the child: And granting the *Fœtus* to be dead, other methods are much more effectual. He was ignorant of the forceps. When the head is left in the *Uterus*, he advises us to extract it, by introducing over it a broad fillet, like a sling.

He is so full on the diseases, that *Boerhaave* recommended him and *Mercatus* to his scholars, on that subject. In his theory of conception, he hath not deviated from the opinions of *Hippocrates*; and in his second volume, he hath published a great many judicious aphorisms, that are now translated into *English* by Mr. *Jones*: Indeed his writings were so universally approved, that they have been translated into several different languages.

Cotemporary with *Mauriceau* were Dr. *Chamberlain* and his three sons, who practised Midwifery in *London* with great reputation. One of these three sons, father to the late Dr. *Hugh Chamberlain*, translated the first

first volume of *Mauriceau* into *English*; and in a note upon that author's method cf extracting the child by the help of the crochet and tire-tête, affirms, that his father, brothers, and himself, were in possession of a much better contrivance for that purpose.

This was no other than the forceps, which they kept as a nostrum, and was not generally known till the year 1733, when a description of the instrument was published by *Chapman*. Long before that, indeed, several kinds of forceps, or extractors, different from those mentioned by the *Arabians*, were used in *France*, *Germany*, and other places; but all of them fell short of the instrument used by the *Chamberlains*, and said to be contrived by the uncle.

In the last century, although there were such excellent practitioners in *London*, and even before the translation of *Mauriceau*, *Guillemeau*'s book on Midwifery had been translated into *English*; and in it all the absurd notions about spells and amulets were left

left out: Neverthelefs, one *Nicholas Culpepper*, who ftiles himfelf gent. ftudent in phyfick and aftronomy, publifhed at *London*, a book intitled, *A Directory for Midwives*; in which he has copied the theory and practice of the old writers, many of whom he mentions, namely, *Hippocrates*, *Galen*, *Ætius*, &c. and frequently advifes the reader to confult his tranflations of *Sennertus*, *Riverius*, *Riolanus*, *Bartholin*, *Johnfton*, *Veflingius*, *Rulandus*, *Sanctor*, *Cole*, the *London Difpenfatory*, and a book which he himfelf had publifhed under the title of *The Englifh Phyfician*. His performances were for many years in great vogue with the midwives, and are ftill read by the lower fort, whofe heads are weak enough to admit fuch ridiculous notions.

He was fucceeded in that way of writing by one Dr. *Salmon*, who was alfo a great tranflator and compiler. He was partly author of a fpurious piece called *Ariftotle's Midwifery*, which hath undergone a great many editions, and contributed to keep up the

the belief of the marvellous effects of various medicines.

Mauriceau, in 1706, publiſhed a ſecond volume, containing about 800 obſervations; but long before that period, he had gained ſuch reputation by his writings, as encouraged others of the ſame nation to write on the ſame ſubject: Accordingly we have the works of *Portal*, *Peu*, and *Dionis*; but all of them fall ſhort of *Mauriceau*. About this time alſo, *Savoiard* wrote ſeveral obſervations on the ſame art.

Henry Daventer practiſed at *Dort*, in *Holland*, and in 1701, publiſhed a book on Midwifery. He obſerved, that an imaginary ſtreight line falling down from the navel, would paſs through the middle of the *Pelvis*: This will nearly hold true, when the *Abdomen* is not diſtended; but in the laſt month of uterine geſtation, in order to paſs through the middle of the *Pelvis*, ſuch a line muſt be let fall from the middle ſpace, betwixt the navel and *Scrobiculum cordis*. This, however,

however, was a good hint, and uſeful in practice.

He pretends to have made ſeveral uſeful diſcoveries, which ſeem feaſible enough to thoſe who have not had the opportunity of an extenſive practice; ſuch as the ſide or wrong poſitions of the *Os internum*, and *Fundus uteri*, which (according to him) are chiefly the occaſion of lingering, difficult, and dangerous labours: He ſeems to have been led into miſtake, by ſuppoſing that the *Placenta* always adhered to the *Fundus uteri*. As to the difficulties proceeding from the wrong poſition of the *Os internum*, a practitioner would, be apt to believe he had never waited for the effect of the labour-pains, which generally open it, by puſhing down the waters, or head of the child.

He was ſeldom called, except in difficult caſes, often proceeding from a diſtorted *Pelvis*, which is common in *Holland*. When this is the caſe, the head of the child is commonly caſt forwards over the *Pubis*, by the jetting in of the *Sacrum*: Or if one *Ilium* is higher

higher than the other, the *Os internum* and *Fundus* are thrown to different ſides; but even then the chief difficulty is owing to the narrowneſs of the *Pelvis*. The *Uterus* is very ſeldom turned ſo oblique as he ſuppoſes it to be; or if it were, provided the child is not too large, nor the *Pelvis* narrow, I never found thoſe difficulties he ſeems to have met with: And ſhould the labour prove tedious, on account of a pendulous belly, by altering the woman's poſition, the obſtacle is commonly removed.

For example: Let her breech be raiſed higher than her ſhoulders; or ſhe may be laid upon her ſide, in a præternatural caſe, when it is neceſſary to turn and deliver the child by the feet. Neverthelefs, though he has run into extremes about the wrong poſitions of the *Uterus*, in which he is the more excuſable, as he had the fondneſs of a parent for a theory that he alledges was his own, yet there are ſome very uſeful hints in his book, particularly that about floodings; in which he directs us to break the membranes, in order

der to reſtrain the *Hæmorrhage*; and his method of dilating the *Os externum*.

The next noted writer in this way, is *Lamotte*, who lived at *Valognes*, near *Caen* in *Normandy*; and in 1715 publiſhed a book on Midwifery, which ſeems to be the beſt of the kind ſince *Mauriceau*, and is tranſlated into *Engliſh* by Mr. *Tomkyns*. It contains about 400 obſervations, the greateſt part of which are illuſtrated with many judicious reflections.

In deſcribing a caſe in which the head preſented, he mentions the great fatigue it had coſt him to turn and deliver by the feet; and hopes that ſome eaſier method will be found out, for extracting the child in ſuch circumſtances: So that, although he wrote ſo lately, he muſt have been ignorant of the forceps. He, as well as *Daventer*, exclaims againſt the uſe of inſtruments; and in moſt laborious caſes, when the head preſented, turned and extracted the *Fœtus* by the feet.

A

A number of ſuch caſes he has recounted; but I am afraid that, like other writers, he has concealed thoſe that would have been more uſeful to the young practitioner, and only given a detail of his own that were ſucceſsful: For certain it is, the head of the child is often ſo large, or the *Pelvis* ſo narrow, that labour-pains cannot poſſibly force it away; and frequently, when the *Fœtus* hath been turned with great fatigue, and the body actually extracted, the force required to deliver the head with the hands alone, is ſuch as deſtroys the child; and ſometimes it is abſolutely impoſſible to bring it along without the help of inſtruments.

For my own part, when I firſt began to practiſe, I determined to follow the method of thoſe gentlemen; but having by theſe means loſt ſeveral children, and ſometimes the mother, I began to alter my opinion, and conſult my own reaſon: In conſequence of which, in caſes of ſuch emergency, I opened the head, with a view of ſaving the woman, if I could not preſerve the life of the child.

In

In the courſe of my deliberations on this ſubject, I likewiſe tried to improve upon the forceps, which ſeemed to me an inſtrument more mechanically adapted, and eaſier applied than any other contrivance hitherto uſed: And ſurely experience juſtifies the uſe of this expedient, by which we are enabled to ſave many children, which otherwiſe muſt have been deſtroyed.

Not that I would be thought to exult over thoſe authors whom I have mentioned, as moſtly enemies to all inſtruments whatever: In other things they have written very judiciouſly, and are blame-worthy in nothing ſo much, as in having ſuppreſſed thoſe unſucceſsful caſes which muſt have happened to men of their extenſive practice.

I own, indeed, when the woman has not ſtrength nor pains ſufficient to force along the child, and the difficulty does not proceed from a large head or narrow *Pelvis*, the method of turning will prove ſucceſsful; but if in the other extreme, I appeal to all candid practitioners, whether many children are not lost, even when the head does not present, and when the body is first brought down, because the *Fœtus* cannot be delivered in another manner.

The next writer in Midwifery is Mr. *Amand* of *Paris*, who describes the method of extracting the head, when left in the *Uterus*, by means of a net. The contrivance is ingenious, but is not applied without great trouble, and cannot succeed when the *Pelvis* is too narrow, or the head too large to pass.

Edmund Chapman practised Midwifery several years in the country, before he settled in *London*; where, in 1733, he published a short account of the practice of midwifery, illustrated with about fifty cases; and is the first person who made publick a description of the forceps used by the *Chamberlains*. *Giffard*'s observations were published in the following year, by Dr. *Hody*, containing many useful remarks and histories of cases in in which he had uſed the extractors or forceps.

Heiſter, profeſſor at *Helmſtadt*, a little town in the dukedom of *Brunſwick*, in the year 1739 publiſhed at *Amſterdam*, a treatiſe on ſurgery; in which we find a very conciſe and diſtinct account of the practice of Midwifery, as well as of the *Cæſarean* operation.

Mr. *Ould*, ſurgeon in *Dublin*, in the year 1742, publiſhed a treatiſe on the practice of Midwifery, in which there are two good obſervations: One relating to a caſe in which the head preſents; and the other ſpecifying what is to be done, when delivery is retarded by the twiſting of the *Funis* round the neck of the child. He prefers his *Terebra oculta* to the ſciſſars, probably becauſe he did not know the proper dimenſions of this laſt inſtrument. The very next year, *Meſnard* publiſhed, at *Paris*, a book on the ſame ſubject, by way of queſtion and anſwer; and is the firſt who contrived the curved, in lieu of the ſtreight crotchets, which is a real improvement.

Over and above the writings of thoſe authors whom I have mentioned, there are a great many curious and extraordinary obſervations on the practice of this art, in *Schenkius*, *Hildanus*, *Bonetus*, the *Philoſophical Tranſactions*, the Academies of Sciences and of Surgeons, and the medical eſſays of *Edinburgh*: And beſides theſe, the beſt modern authors who have written on the diſeaſes of women and children, are *Sydenham*, *Harris*, *Boerhaave*, *Friend*, *Hamilton*, *Hoffman*, and *Shaw*.

On the whole, that the young practitioner may not be miſled by the uſeleſs theories, and uncertain conjectures of both antient and modern writers, it may be neceſſary to obſerve in general, that all the hypotheſes hitherto eſpouſed, are liable to many material objections; and that almoſt every ſyſtem hath been overthrown by that which followed it.

This

This will, probably, be always the caſe; and, indeed, as theory is but of little ſervice towards aſcertaining the diagnoſtics and cure of diſeaſes, or improving the practice of Midwifery, ſuch enquiries are the leſs material. What *Hippocrates* has written about the form of the *Uterus*, and its various motions, conception, the formation of the child, the ſeventh and eighth month's births, was, till the laſt century, believed as infallible aſſertions; when his doctrine of conception, and the nutrition of the *Fœtus* was overthrown; and many new and uncertain theories, on the ſame ſubject, introduced.

Some of the moderns conclude, that the antients never turned and brought children by the feet, becauſe *Hippocrates* directs us, in all caſes, to bring the head into the natural ſituation; and ſays, that when delivery is performed by the feet, both mother and child are in imminent danger. *Celſus*, and all the writers till the time of *Paræus*, adopted this practice of bringing the head to preſent: But, at the ſame time, many of them obſerve, that if this be not practicable, we muſt ſearch for the feet, and deliver the *Fœtus* in that manner. *Celſus* ſays, if the feet are at hand, the child is eaſily delivered footling: And *Philomenus* goes ſtill farther, ſaying, that if even the head ſhould preſent, and the child cannot be delivered in that poſition, we muſt turn and bring it by the feet.

With regard to the fillets and forceps, they have been alledged to be late inventions; yet we find *Avicenna* recommending the uſe of both: And although, by the figures of the forceps given by *Albucaſis*, who repreſents them furniſhed with long ſharp teeth, one would imagine the inſtrument was deſigned for ſqueezing the bones, and bringing the child along at any rate, without endeavouring to ſave its life, yet the forceps recommended by *Avicen*, is plainly intended to ſave the *Fœtus*; for he ſays, if it cannot be extracted by this inſtrument, the head muſt be opened, and the ſame method uſed, which he deſcribes in

his

his chapter on the delivery of dead children.

To conclude, we find among the ancients ſeveral valuable jewels, buried under the rubbiſh of ignorance and ſuperſtition; becauſe the aſſiſtance of men was ſeldom ſolicited in caſes of Midwifery, till the laſt extremity: And thoſe diſadvantages being conſidered, we ought to be ſurpriſed at finding ſo many excellent obſervations in the courſe of their practice; and be aſhamed of ourſelves for the little improvement we have made in ſo many centuries, notwithſtanding our opportunities, and the advantages we had from their experience.

True it is, we have eſtabliſhed a better method of delivering in laborious and præternatural caſes; by which many children are ſaved, that muſt have been deſtroyed by their manner of practice: but are not many of our modern practitioners juſtly branded for their ſordid and unſocial principles, in profeſſing noſtrums, both with regard to medicines and methods of delivery? Infomuch, that I have heard a gentleman of eminence in one of the branches of medicine affirm, that he never knew one perfon of our profeffion, who did not pretend to be in poffeffion of fome fecret or another: From whence he concluded, that we were altogether a body of empirics. Such reflections ought to make a fuitable impreffion upon the minds of the honeft and ingenuous, prompt them to lay afide all fuch pitiful, felfifh confiderations, and, for the future, act with opennefs and candour; which cannot fail of redounding to the honour of the profeffion, and the good of fociety, as well as their own advantage.

BOOK I.

CHAP. I.

The structure and form of the Pelvis, *so far as it is necessary to be known in the practice of Midwifery.*

SECT. I.

Of the BONES.

THE *Pelvis* is composed of three bones; the *Os sacrum*, with its appendix, known by the name of *Coccyx*, and the two *Ossa innominata*. The *Sacrum* in children is divided into five distinct bones, and the *Coccyx* into four cartilages; but in adults, these last are formed into as many moveable

bones,

bones, and the divisions of the *Sacrum* ossified so as to become one bone.

Each *Os innominatum* is, in infants, composed of three different bones, under the appellation of *Ilium*, *Ischium*, and *Pubis*; which are joined to one another at the *Acetabulum*, or cavity, that receives the round head of the thigh-bone. This composition is, in point of figure, so irregular, that although in adults the three are ossified into one bone, those different names are still used, in order to distinguish one part of it from the other.

The *Ossa innominata* of the opposite sides are joined to one another in the fore-part, at the *Pubis*, by a thick cartilage and strong ligaments; and the posterior part of each *Os ilium* is connected with the upper and lateral part of the *Sacrum* by the same apparatus.

Divers authors and practitioners in this art have alledged, that towards the latter end of gestation, when all the parts of the *Abdomen* are strongly pressed by the increased *Uterus*, an extraordinary quantity of *Mucus* is secreted, not only by the glands of the *Os*

in-

internum and *Vagina*, but alſo by thoſe belonging to the cartilages and ligaments, that connect the bones of the *Pelvis*; by which means, the ligaments and cartilages are ſoftened and relaxed, and the bones are ſeparated from one another in time of labour: But from experience and obſervation I may venture to aſſert, that this ſeparation is by no means an uſual ſymptom, though ſometimes it may happen; in which caſe the patient ſuffers great pain, and continues lame in thoſe parts for a conſiderable time after delivery.

In ſome women, indeed, a kind of obſcure motion may be perceived, when the child's head is forced into the *Pelvis*, by ſtrong pains: The junctures of the *Sacrum* with the *Ilia*, as well as that of the *Oſſa pubis*, ſeem to yield a very little alternately, in order to accommodate themſelves to the ſhape of the head, as it is ſqueezed down and paſſes along through the *Pelvis*; but the bones are not ſeparated to any conſiderable diſtance.

The *Coccyx* is moveable at its connection with the *Sacrum*; as are alſo the four bones that

that compoſe it, in their articulations one with another; and this motion continues in adults, as well as in thoſe of more tender years: In old age, indeed, and even in young people who have ſuffered bruiſes upon the part, attended with great pain and inflammation, we frequently find the different pieces of this bone rigidly cemented together: But this *Anchyloſis* the more ſeldom happens, becauſe they undergo a gentle motion at every excretion of the *Fæces*, which helps to preſerve their mobility.

SECT. II.

THE brim or upper part of a well-ſhap'd *Pelvis* repreſents a kind of imperfect oval, or ſomething that approaches a triangular figure: If we conſider it as an oval, the long axis paſſes from ſide to ſide; but as a triangle, the poſterior part forms one ſide, and the *Pubis* conſtitutes the oppoſite angle; ſo that behind it is compoſed of the broad part of the *Sacrum*, where it joins with the laſt *Vertebra* of the loins; on each ſide by the inferior parts of the *Ilia*; and

and before, by the ſuperior parts of the *Oſſa pubis*.

The lower circumference of the *Pelvis* is formed, behind, by the inferior part of the *Sacrum* and its appendage; on each ſide, by the lower part of each *Iſchium* and a broad ligament which riſes from the ſpine of that bone, and, with the *Coccigæus* muſcle, is inſerted into the edge of the *Coccyx* and the lower part of the *Sacrum*; and before, by the inferior parts of the *Oſſa pubis* and the two proceſſes that deſcend on each ſide, to join with thoſe that riſe from the *Iſchia*; by which conjunction the *Framen Magnum Iſchii*, is formed on each ſide.

When the body of a woman is reclined backwards, or half-ſitting, half-lying, the brim of the *Pelvis* is horizontal, and an imaginary ſtreight line deſcending from the navel, would paſs through the middle of the cavity; but in the laſt month of pregnancy, ſuch a line muſt take its riſe from the middle ſpace between the navel and *Scrobiculum cordis*, in order to paſs through the ſame point of the *Pelvis*.

SECT.

SECT. III.

IN the consideration of the *Pelvis*, three circumstances are to be principally regarded and remembered; namely, the width, the depth, and form of the cavity on the inside.

1. The extent of the brim from the back to the forepart, commonly amounts to four inches and one quarter; and from one side to the other, the distance is five inches and a quarter: So that this difference of an inch in the different axes, ought to be carefully attended to in the practice of Midwifery. But the width of the lower part of the *Pelvis* is the reverse of this calculation, when the *Os coccygis* is pressed backward by the head of the child: because in that case, the distance between the *Coccyx* and the lower part of the *Pubis*, is five inches and a quarter; whereas the inferior and posterior parts of one *Os ischium*, are no more than four inches and a quarter, from the same parts of the other. Indeed the width of the lower part of the *Pelvis* is naturally the same, in both diameters; so that this dif-

difference of an inch is occaſioned by the yielding of the *Coccyx* in the birth.

2. The depth of the *Pelvis*, from the upper part of the *Sacrum*, where it is articulated with the laſt *Vertebra* of the loins, to the lower end of the *Coccyx*, is about five inches in a ſtreight line; but when this appendix is ſtretched outward and backward, the diſtance will be one inch more.

The depth from the ſides of the brim towards its fore-part, to the lower parts of the *Iſchia*, is four inches; and from the upper to the lower parts of the *Oſſa pubis*, where they join, the diſtance is no more than two inches: So that in the dimenſions of the *Pelvis*, the ſide is twice, and the back part three times the depth of the forepart.

3. Nor is the form and ſhape of the inſide of the *Pelvis* to be neglected by the practitioners of Midwifery.

The *Sacrum* and *Coccyx* being convex on the outſide, exhibit a concave figure on the inſide; the curve being increaſed towards the lower end, ſo as that from the extremity of the *Coccyx* to the middle of the *Sacrum*, the ſweep nearly repreſents a ſemicircle;

and from thence the bone ſlopes upward and forward.

From the upper part of the brim on each ſide, (but nearer the fore than the back part) to the lower parts of the *Iſchia*, the deſcent is perpendicular: And the opening on each ſide, betwixt the lower parts of the *Sacrum* and the poſterior part of each *Iſchium*, is about three inches deep, and two and an half in width. The upper part of this vacuity on each ſide, gives paſſage and lodgement to a muſcle, veſſels, nerves, *&c.* At its lower part, the *Coccygæus* muſcle and ligament above mentioned, are ſtretched acroſs from bone to bone; and this ligament is on the outſide ſtrengthened with another ſtrong expanſion, riſing from the tuberoſity of the *Iſchium*, and fixed into the edge of the *Sacrum* and *Coccyx*. All theſe parts yield and ſtretch, forming a concave equal to that of the *Sacrum*, when the fore or hind-head of the child is puſhed down at the ſide and back part of the *Pelvis*.

From the upper to the under-parts of the *Oſſa pubis*, which form the anterior angle of the *Pelvis*, the deſcent is almoſt perpendicular,

dicular, or rather inclining a little forwards: So that on the whole, the inſide of the baſin is bent downwards into a concave behind, and deſcends in a ſtreight line before; while the *Ilia* ſlope outwards as they riſe, and the *Vertebræ* of the loins turn backwards, making an obtuſe angle with the *Sacrum*.

On the whole, it is of the utmoſt conſequence to know, that the brim of the *Pelvis* is wider from ſide to ſide, than from the back to the forepart; but that at the under part of the baſin, the dimenſions are the reverſe of this proportion; and that the back-part, in point of depth, is to the fore-part as three to one, and to the ſides as three to two.

Though thoſe dimenſions obtain in a well-ſhaped *Pelvis*, they ſometimes vary in different women; and the reaſon of this remark will be more fully explained, when we treat of the method of delivery, in the different kinds of labours.

SECT. IV.

Of a diſtorted PELVIS.

THE *Pelvis*, in decrepit women, is not always diſtorted, becauſe the diſtortion of the ſpine, in many women, does not happen till the age of eight, ten, twelve, or fourteen; when, being tall and ſlender, it is occaſioned by miſmanagement in their dreſs, lying too much on one ſide, and other accidents; without having any effect upon the *Pelvis*, the ſhape of which is by that time aſcertained.

But moſt of thoſe who have been ricketty in their infancy, whether they continue little and deformed, or, recovering of that diſeaſe, grow up to be tall ſtately women, are commonly narrow and diſtorted in the *Pelvis*; and conſequently ſubject to tedious and difficult labours: For, as the *Pelvis* is more or leſs diſtorted, the labour is more or leſs dangerous and difficult.

In ricketty children, the bones are ſoft and flexible; and as they cannot run about and exerciſe themſelves like thoſe of a more hardy make, the *Pelvis*, in ſitting upon ſtools or the nurſe's knees, is by the weight of the head and body, often bent and diſtorted in the following manner:

The *Coccyx* and lower part of the *Sacrum* are preſſed inward and backward, and the extremity of the *Coccyx* bent too much forward

ward towards the under part of the *Pubis*; and when the lower part of the *Sacrum* is preſſed upward and outward, the ſuperior part is turned forward with the laſt *Vertebra* of the loins, approaching too near to the upper part of the *Pubis*: So that the diſtance in ſome women, from the back to the fore-part of the brim, is not above three inches; in others, no more than two; and ſometimes, though rarely, not above one inch and an half.

In others, the lower *Vertebra* of the loins, with the upper end of the *Sacrum* jet inwards and to one ſide: The *Pubis*, inſtead of being inwardly concave, is ſometimes convex; and the lower part of each *Iſchium* ſo near to one another, that the diſtance, inſtead of four inches and one quarter, will not amount to more than three, and in ſome caſes not ſo much.

Sometimes the *Vertebræ* that compoſe the *Sacrum* ride one another, and form a large protuberance in that part which ought to be concave; but the moſt common circumſtance of diſtortion, is the jetting forward of the laſt *Vertebra* of the loins with the upper end of the *Sacrum*, forming a more acute angle with the ſpine; and in this part of the paſſage the head moſt commonly ſticks.

SECT. V.

THE *Pelvis* in women is wider than in men, the *Ilia* ſpreading more outward, in order to ſuſtain and allow free ſpace for the ſtretching of the *Uterus*; the *Sacrum* is more concave, and the proceſſes of the *Oſſa pubis*, at their junction with the *Iſchia*, are not ſo near to one another; while the breaſt-bones are more flat in women than in men, to make an allowance for the ſuperior ſize of their breaſts.

In order to demonſtrate the advantage of knowing the wideneſs, depth, and figure of the inſide of a well formed *Pelvis*, it will be neceſſary to aſcertain the dimenſions of the head of the child, and the manner of its paſſage in a natural birth.

The heads of thoſe children that have paſſed eaſily through a large *Pelvis*, as well as of thoſe that have been brought by the feet, without having ſuffered any al-

alteration in point of ſhape,. by the uncommon circumſtances of the labour; I ſay, ſuch heads are commonly about an inch narrower from ear to ear, than from the fore to the under-part of the hind-head.

That part of the head which preſents, is not the *Fontanelle* (as was formerly ſuppoſed) but the ſpace between the *Fontanelle* and where the *Lambdoidal* croſſes the end of the *Sagittal ſuture*, and the hair of the ſcalp diverges or goes off on all ſides: For, in moſt laborious caſes, when the head is ſqueezed along with great force, we find it preſſed intc a very oblong form, the longeſt axis of which extends from the face to the *Vertix*. From whence it appears, that the crown or *Vertix* is the firſt part that is preſſed down, becauſe in the general preſſure, the bones at that part of the ſkull make the leaſt reſiſtance, and the face is always turned upward; ſometimes, indeed, this lengthening or protuberance is found at a little diſtance from the *Vertix*, backward or forward, or on either ſide; and ſometimes (though very ſeldom) the *Fontanelle* or forehead preſents; in which caſe they protuberate, while the *Vertix* is preſt, and remains quite flat: But theſe two inſtances do not occur more than once in fifty or an hundred caſes that are laborious.

Now, ſuppoſing the *Vertix* is that part of the head which preſents itſelf to the touch, in the progreſs of its deſcent, the *Fontanelle* is commonly turned more upwards, and to one ſide of the *Pelvis*; and when the hindhead comes down to the *Os iſchium* of the contrary ſide, one may feel the *Lambdoidal ſuture* where it croſſes the end of the *Sagittal*, and, unleſs the ſcalp is very much ſwelled, diſtinguiſh the *Occiput* at its junction with the parietal bones, by the angle, which is more obtuſe than thoſe that are formed on the other parts of the ſkull: Beſides, in this poſition, the ear of the child may be eaſily perceived at the *Pubis*. As the head is forced farther along, the hindhead riſes gradually into the open ſpace below the *Pubis*, which is two inches higher than the *Iſchium*, while, at the ſame time, the forehead turns into the hollow of the *Sacrum*.

This,

This, therefore, is the manner of its progreſſion: When the head firſt preſents itſelf at the brim of the *Pelvis*, the forehead is to one ſide, and the hindhead to the other, and ſometimes it is placed diagonal in the cavity: Thus the wideſt part of the head is turned to the wideſt part of the *Pelvis*, and the narrow part of the head, from ear to ear, applied to the narrow part of the *Pelvis*, between the *Pubis* and the *Sacrum*. The head being ſqueezed along, the *Vertix* deſcends to the lower part of the *Iſchium*; where the *Pelvis* becoming narrower at the ſides, the wide part of the head can proceed no farther in the ſame line of direction: But the *Iſchium* being much lower than the *Pubis*, the hindhead is forced in below this laſt bone, where there is leaſt reſiſtance. The forehead then turns into the hollow at the lower end of the *Sacrum*, and now again the narrow part of the head is turned to the narrow part of the *Pelvis*: The *Os pubis* being only two inches deep, the *Vertix* and hindhead riſe upward from below it; the forehead preſſes back the *Coccyx*, and the head riſing up-

 ward

ward by degrees, comes out with an half round turn from below the ſhare-bone: The wide part of the head being now betwixt the *Pubis* and the *Coccyx*, which being puſhed backwards, opens the wideſt ſpace below, and allows the forehead to riſe up alſo with a half round turn, from the under part of the *Os externum*.

From theſe particulars, any perſon will perceive the advantage of remembering, that the *Pelvis* at the brim is wider from ſide to ſide, than from the fore to the back-part, while below it is the reverſe, in point of dimenſion; that the *Pelvis* is much ſhallower at the *Pubis* than at the ſides and back-part; and that the *Sacrum* and *Coccyx* form a large concave in their deſcent, whereas that of the *Pubis* is perpendicular: Neither is it leſs neceſſary to conſider the form of the head, as above deſcribed; for the knowledge of theſe things will convey a diſtinct idea of the manner in which the head is to be brought along in laborious caſes; on what occaſions the uſe of the forceps may be neceſſary; when the body is delivered before the head; and when the method

muſt

muſt be varied, as the form of the head or *Pelvis* may chance to vary from our deſcription.

Although the poſition of the head, in natural and laborious births, is commonly ſuch as we have obſerved, it is not always the ſame; but ſometimes differs, according to the different figures of the *Pelvis* and head, and the poſture of the child *in utero:* For when the waters are in ſmall quantity, or the membranes broke, ſo that the body of the child is cloſe confined by the womb, if the fore-parts are towards the belly of the mother, that poſition may hinder the head from making the proper turns as it is puſhed down, and the forehead may be forced towards the groin or *Pubis*. Sometimes, even in a well-formed *Pelvis*, if the *Fontanelle* preſents itſelf, with the forehead to one ſide of the brim, and the hindhead to the other, when the head is forced down by the increaſing pains, there will be leſs reſiſtance at the *Vertix* than at any other part; conſequently the diameter from the fore to the hindhead will be leſſened, and this laſt by accommodating itſelf to the circumſtances of the preſſure, be firſt ſqueezed down,

down, and at length come forward in the natural way: Or ſhould the ear preſent itſelf, the *Vertix* will be firſt forced down in the ſame manner. But if the forehead be nearer than the *Vertix* to the middle of the brim of the *Pelvis*, every pain will force it farther down; and, when delivered, it will riſe in form of an obtuſe cone or ſugar-loaf, and in that caſe the crown of the head will be altogether flat. But if inſtead of the *Vertix* or forehead, the *Fontanelle* ſhould firſt appear, the ſpace from the forehead to the crown will then riſe in form of a ſow's back; and in all theſe caſes, the head is brought along with greater difficulty, than in thoſe where the *Vertix* is firſt produced: And in all laborious caſes, the *Vertix* comes down and is lengthened in form of a ſugar-loaf, nine and forty times in fifty inſtances. When the forehead preſents, the face is ſometimes preſſed forwards. If the *Pelvis* be as wide from the back to the forepart, as from ſide to ſide, (though this ſeldom happens) the crown may be puſhed down at the *Pubis*, and the foredead afterwards ſqueezed into the hollow of the

Sacrum, without making the foregoing turns. If the belly of the child is to the forepart of the *Uterus*, the *Vertix* may be towards the *Sacrum*, and the forehead to the *Pubis* or groin: So that all theſe uncommon poſitions are attended with difficulty.

CHAP. II.

Of the external and internal parts of Generation proper to Women.

SECT. I.

The external parts and VAGINA.

THE *Mons Veneris* is ſituated at the upper part of the *Pubis*, from which alſo begin the *Labia pudendi*, ſtretching down as far as the lower edge where the *Frænum labiorum* or *Fourchette* is formed; and here it will not be amiſs to obſerve, that the œdematous ſwelling of the *Labia*, which often happens, is no manner of obſtruction to delivery.

The *Clitoris*, with its *Præputium*, is found between the *Labia* on the middle and fore-

part

part of the *Pubis*; and from the lower part of the *Clitoris*, the *Nymphæ* rising, spread outwards and downwards to the sides of the *Os externum*, forming a kind of *Sulcus* or furrow, called the *Fossa magna* or *Navicularis*, for the direction of the *Penis* in coition, or of the finger in touching, into the *Vagina*.

The *Meatus urinarius* is immediately below the under-edge of the *Symphysis* of the *Ossa pubis*, and at the upper part of the *Os externum*, which is the orifice of the *Vagina*, situated immediately below the said bones of the *Pubis*; the lower edge of which bones is equal to the lower edge of the *Frænum* or *Fourchette*, which bounds the inferior part of the *Fossa magna* and *Os externum*, restraining it as if with a bridle.

The *Perinæum* extends from this border to the *Anus*, being about one inch, or one and an half in length; the wrinkled part of the *Anus* is about three quarters of an inch in diameter; from thence to the *Coccyx* the distance is about two inches; so that the whole extent, from the *Fourchette* to this bone,

bone, amounts to about four inches, or four and a quarter.

What remains of the lower part of the *Pelvis*, is covered and filled up with the integuments, adipoſe membrane, and the muſcles called *Levatores ani*; while within theſe are contained the muſcles belonging to the *Clitoris*, mouth of the bladder, *Os externum*, and *Anus*.

In young children there is a thin membrane called the *Hymen*, extended over the lower part of the *Os externum*, repreſenting the figure of a creſcent; the concave and open ſide being turned towards the *Meatus urinarius*. In ſome the middle of this concave is attached to the lower part of the *Meatus*, forming two ſmall openings on each ſide, which in grown women will ſcarce admit a ſmall probe, unleſs the membrane has been previouſly broke in coition: Nay, in ſome adults this membrane has entirely ſhut up the entrance of the *Vagina*, ſo that they havę been altogether imperforated; but when broke, it recedes and forms the *Carunculæ myrtiformes*.

On

On each ſide of the *Meatus urinarius*, are two ſmall *Lacunæ* or openings, the tubes of which ending in a kind of *Sacculus*, come from the proſtate gland: From theſe a thin fluid is ejected in time of copulation, and that from ſome women with conſiderable force; and ſometimes, though ſeldom, to the quantity of ſeveral drams.

The *Urethra* in women is about one inch and an half in length. The *Vagina* is formed of a ſtrong, thick membrane, of a ſpungy texture, more contracted in virgins than in married women. When ſtretched to its full extent, it may be about five, ſix, or ſeven inches long, and two in width, according to the difference of ſtature in different women; but when the *Uterus* hangs down in the *Vagina*, the length will not be more than two or three inches; and it may be ſtretched with the finger to the wideneſs of three or four. The inſide of it in young women, is full of *rugæ*, folds or wrinkles, which are partly obliterated in thoſe who have bore children: The upper end of the *Vagina* is joined to the circumference of the lips of the *Os uteri*, which

which reſemble the mouth of a puppy or tench; and a thin expanſion of this membrane being reflected inwards, covers the exterior part of theſe lips, which in virgins are ſmooth and of an oval form: It is alſo continued along the inſide of the *Uterus*, conſtituting the internal membrane of the neck and *Fundus*, which is likewiſe full of *Plicæ*, eſpecially in young ſubjects.

As to the different names of thoſe parts, the book of *Schurigius*, publiſhed at *Dreſden* in the year 1729, may be conſulted. The entry of the *Vagina* is commonly called the *Sphincter vaginæ*, and the mouth of the womb is often diſtinguiſhed by the appellation of *Os tincæ*: but as the mention of theſe parts will frequently occur in the courſe of this treatiſe, I ſhall, in order to avoid confuſion or miſtake, call the firſt *Os externum*, and the other *Os internum*, through the whole book.

SECT.

SECT. II.

Of the UTERUS.

THE *Uterus* is about three inches long, from the *Os internum* to the upper part of the *Fundus*, and one inch in thickneſs from the fore to the back-part. It is divided into the neck and *Fundus*, the length of the neck being an inch and three quarters, while that of the *Fundus* is one inch and one quarter. The width of the *Uterus* at the neck is about one inch, but at the *Fundus*, twice as much. The *Uterus* is ſmaller in young women.

The outſide ſhape of the *Uterus*, in ſome meaſure, reſembes a flattened cucurbit, or that kind of pear which hath a long neck.

The canal or entrance from the *Os internum* to the cavity of the *Fundus uteri*, will admit a common director; being a little wider in the middle and more contracted at the upper end.

The cavity of the *Fundus* is, in point of figure, ſomething between an oval and triangle; one of the angles commencing at the upper end of the foreſaid canal, and the

the other two expanding the ſides of the *Fundus*, from which ariſe the Fallopian tubes. Theſe tubes or trumpets are about three inches long, and ſo narrow at their entrance from the *Uterus*, as ſcarcely to admit an hog's briſtle; but the cavity of each turns gradually wider, and ends in an open mouth or ſphincter, from the brim of which is expanded the *Fimbria* or *Morſus diaboli*, that generally bears the likeneſs of jagged leaves, and in ſome reſembles an hand with membranous fingers, which is ſuppoſed to graſp the *Ovum* when ripe and ready to drop from the *Ovarium*.

The *Uterus* is formed, firſt of the inſide membrane that riſes from the *Vagina*, and lines all the interior part of the womb: Immediately above this coat is the thick ſubſtance of the *Uterus*, compoſed of a *Plexus* of arteries, lymphaticks, veins and nerves, and the veſſels on its ſurface, when injected, ſeem to run in contorted lines. It appears to be of the ſame glandular texture (though not ſo compact) as that of the *Mamma* in the breaſts, without any muſcular fibres, except ſuch as compoſe the coats of the veſſels: neither is there any neceſſity for that muſcle which *Ruych* pretended to diſcover at the *Fundus*, for the convenience of forcing off the *Placenta*; becauſe this cake as frequently adheres to other parts of the womb as to the *Fundus*.

The ſubſtance of the *Uterus* appears more compact and pale than that of muſcles; or, if it be muſcular, at leaſt the fibres are more cloſe, and more intricately diſpoſed, than in other muſcular parts. The blood veſſels of the womb, in the virgin or unimpregnated ſtate, are very ſmall, except juſt at their approach to its ſides, at the roots of the *Ligamenta lata*; but as ſoon almoſt as they enter its ſubſtance, they are diſperſed into ſuch numbers of ſmaller branches through the whole, that when it is cut, we can obſerve but few, and thoſe very ſmall orifices, much leſs any cavities that deſerve the name of *Sinuſes*. Indeed, when this part is minutely injected, it ſeems to be almoſt nothing but a maſs of veſſels; a circumſtance common to it, with other parts of the body: And anatomiſts are agreed, that the greater number of veſſels viſible in ſuch nice injections,

tions, are thoſe through which the ſerum or lymph of the blood circulate in the living body; whence the *Error loci* in an *Opthalmia*, is imitated by ſubtile injections of coloured matter into the arteries of the dead ſubject.

When the *Uterus* ſtretches in time of geſtation, the veſſels are proportionably dilated by an increaſe of the fluid they contain; ſo that, at the time of delivery, ſome of them are capacious enough to admit the end of the little finger. Yet the ſubſtance of the womb, inſtead of growing thinner, as *Mauriceau* alledges, or thicker, according to *Daventer*, continues of its natural thickneſs during the whole term of pregnancy; and this equality is maintained by the gradual diſtenſion of the veſſels that enter into its compoſition. In time of labour, indeed, as the waters are diſcharged, the *Uterus* contracts itſelf and grows thicker; and the reſiſtance ceaſing at the delivery of the child and after-birth, it becomes ſmaller and ſmaller, until it has nearly reſumed its natural dimenſions.

For as the *Uterus* contracts itſelf after parturition, the arterial blood cannot flow into it in the ſame quantity as that with which the veſſels were filled in their ſtate of diſtention. The fluids are gradually emptied into the *Vena cava aſcendens*, but chiefly through the mouths of the veſſels that open into the cavity of the womb; and the veſſels themſelves that were ſtretched, elongated, and ſeemed to recede from one another, are alſo contracted by degrees, and that in ſuch a direction, as to reduce the *Uterus* into the ſame ſhape and ſize which it bore before impregnation: Nay, the fibres are again ſo compacted, that they, and even the veſſels, are ſcarce diſcernable.

The *Vagina* on its out-ſide is covered with a thick adipoſe membrane: by means of which it is on the forepart attached to the lower part of the bladder, and on the back part to the lower end of the *Rectum* and *Anus*; and by the ſame means all theſe parts are connected with the *Peritoneum*, or internal ſurface of the *Pelvis*.

The *Uterus* is contained in a duplicature of the *Peritoneum*, which covers it every where

where above, and is connected with its ſubſtance by a very thin cellular membrane; as for the *Peritoneum* in itſelf, it is a ſmooth membranous expanſion, that covers all the inſide of the *Abdomen*, and gives external coats to all the *Viſcera* contained in that cavity. On the fore-part, it lines the muſcles of the *Abdomen* and *Diaphragm*; backwards, it covers the abdominal *Viſcera* in general, the *Aorta* and *Vena cava deſcendens*, the kidneys, ureters, and ſpermatick veſſels, the external and internal *Iliacs*, the *Pſoas* and muſcles that cover the inſide of the *Ilium*; whence it riſes double, and forms the *Ligamenta lata*, in which are contained the *Ovaria* and Fallopian tubes. This duplicature, where it meets in the middle, invelops all the *Uterus*, as before obſerved, and gives a covering to the round ligaments that riſe from each ſide of the *Fundus uteri*, and are inſerted or loſt about the upper and external part of the *Pubis* and groin. The *Peritoneum* is alſo reflected from the forepart of the *Uterus*, over the upper-part of the bladder; and upon the back-part of the *Uterus*, it deſcends even upon the *Vagina*, from which it is again reflected upwards over the *Rectum*. By theſe attachments, eſpecially the broad and round ligaments, the *Uterus* is kept between the *Veſica urinaria* and *rectum*, looſely ſuſpended in the *Vagina*, within two or three inches of the *Os externum*; the *Os internum* being turned back in the lower part of the *Vagina*, towards the *Anus* or lower part of the *Rectum*; ſituated in the courſe of the ſtreight line, paſſing through the middle of the *Pelvis*. In coition, the *Uterus* yields three or four inches to the preſſure of the *Penis*, having a free motion upwards and downwards, ſo that the reciprocal oſcillation which is permitted by this contrivance, increaſes the mutual titillation and pleaſure.

The ligaments undergo no extraordinary extenſion in time of uterine geſtation, becauſe they ſink down two inches with the *Uterus* in an unimpregnated ſtate; and when the *Fundus* riſes, they will be raiſed at the ſame time, to the height of not only theſe two inches, but as much more, without being ſtretched in the leaſt: Beſides, as the *Uterus* riſes ſtill upwards, the ſides of it

ap-

approach the *Ilia*, from whence the broad ligaments take their origin, and this circumſtance is equal to an acquiſition of three inches more; ſo that upon the whole, theſe ligaments ſeem to be very little ſtretched, even in the laſt month of pregnancy.

SECT. III.

Of the Ovaria, *veſſels, ligaments, and Fallopian tubes.*

THE *Ovaria* are two ſmall oval bodies, one of which is placed behind each Fallopian tube; ſuppoſed to be little more than a cluſter of *Ova*, whence they derive their preſent name: for by ancient authors they are mentioned by the appellation of the female teſticles. Each *Ovarium* is about one inch in length, half as broad, and one quarter of an inch in thickneſs; more convex on the fore than on the back part, of a ſmooth ſurface, covered with the *Peritoneum*.

The blood veſſels are, firſt, the ſpermatick arteries and veins, which have nearly the ſame origin as thoſe in men, are moſtly di-

diſtributed upon the *Ovaria* and tubes, and at the upper part of the *Uterus* communicate with the hypogaſtricks, from the branches of which the body of the womb is furniſhed. All theſe arteries anaſtomoſe, and are ſuppoſed to detach ſmall ramifications that open into the cavity of the *Uterus*. The veins are large, communicate one with another, with the *Hæmorrhoidals* and *Vena portarum*, and have no valves.

The *Ligamenta rotunda* are two vaſcular ropes, compoſed of veins and arteries incloſed in the duplicature of the *Ligamenta lata*; ſeemingly ariſing from the crural artery and vein, from whence they are extended to the ſides of the *Fundus uteri*.

The nerves come from the intercoſtals, *Lumbares*, and *Sacri*; as deſcribed in *Boerhaave*'s inſtitutes, and *Winſlow*'s anatomy.

CHAP.

CHAP. III.

SECT. I.

Of the CATAMENIA *and* FLUOR ALBUS, *in an unimpregnated ſtate.*

THE *Uterus*, according to ſome, and all the parts ſubſervient to generation, arrive at full growth about the age of fifteen: The veſſels are then ſufficiently dilated, and thoſe that end in the cavity of the womb ſo diſtended with blood, that their ſphincters or mouths are forced open, they empty themſelves gradually, and for that time the *Plethora* in the *Uterus* and neighbouring parts is removed.

Several ingenious theories have been erected, to account for the flux of the *Menſes*; particularly by Doctors *Friend*, *Simpſon*, and *Aſtruc*, the two laſt of whom, with many others, alledge, that there are *Sinuſes* in the *Uterus*, furniſhed with ſide-veſſels opening into its cavity; which *Sinuſes* are gradually ſtretched by the blood they receive from the ar-

arteries, until the fourth or beginning of the fifth week, the lateral veſſels are forced open, and the accumulated blood evacuated into the cavity of the womb. But if this were the caſe, the ſame mechaniſm muſt prevail in other parts of the body, through which the like periodical diſcharge is made, when the *Uterus* is obſtructed; as from the noſe, hairy ſcalp, lungs, ſtomach, meſenteric and hæmorrhoidal veſſels, and even through the ſkin of the legs, and other parts of the body. Beſides, ſuch an accumulation in large *Sinuſes*, though the blood were not entirely ſtagnated, would produce a viſcoſity like that which obtains in rheumatiſms and other inflammatory diſtempers.

Thoſe who live in hot climates, are frequently viſited with the *Menſes* at the age of twelve; and women who are kept warm, and live delicately, undergo this diſcharge earlier than thoſe who uſe a different regimen: And if the *Catamenia* do not flow at the ſtated time, the patient is ſoon after ſeized with the *Chloroſis*, unleſs ſome other evacuation happens in lieu of the *Menſes*.

They

They commonly ceaſe to flow about the age of forty-five, except in thoſe with whom they began at twelve, or in ſuch as have born a great many children; in which caſe they ceaſe about the age of two and forty, or ſooner.

In young people the *Momentum* of the circulating fluid is greater than the reſiſting force of the ſolids; ſo that the veſſels continue to be gradually ſtretched, until, by their number, capacity, and length, this *Momentum* is diſſipated, ſo as to become no more than equal to the reſiſtance. About this time the ſuperplus of blood begins to be diſcharged, and thus the *Æquilibrium* is preſerved till the age of forty five; when the fibres growing rigid, the *Incrementum* is leſſened, the evacuation is no longer neceſſary, nor has the blood force enough to make good its wonted paſſage into the cavity of the womb. In the ſame manner are produced the ſymptoms of old age.

The *Catamenia* are, therefore, no more than a periodical diſcharge of that ſuperplus of blood, which is collected through the month, and, towards the criſis, attended with pains in the loins, breaſt, and head, more or leſs acute, according to the circumſtances of the *Plethora*; all which complaints gradually vaniſh when the *Menſes* begin to appear.

This evacuation commonly continues till the fifth or ſixth day, in ſome to the third only, and in others to the ſeventh: The quantity diſcharged being, according to *Hippocrates*, two *hemina*, equal, by the computation of ſome, to eighteen or twenty, and, in the opinion of others, to twenty-four ounces: but this muſt certainly be a miſtake; for they rarely exceed four ounces, except when they flow in too great quantity.

Women that are delicately kept, and plentifully fed, have this diſcharge more frequently, and in greater quantity, than thoſe who are inured to much exerciſe, or ſubject to copious perſpiration; yet both theſe conſtitutions may be healthy, and ought not to be tampered with by preſcriptions for altering the period or quantity of this evacuation. Indeed, if the flux be ſo frequent or immoderate as to exhauſt the ſtrength of the patient, it will be neceſſary to preſcribe bleeding

ing before the return of the period, reſt, cooling and aſtringent medicines, not only taken internally, but likewiſe applied externally, and injected into the *Vagina.*

On the contrary, if they flow too ſeldom, in too ſmall quantity, or do not appear at all, ſo that a dangerous plenitude enſues, the *Plethora* muſt be leſſened by plentiful bleeding and repeated purges, and the diſcharge ſollicited by warm baths, fumigation, and exerciſe. But if the patient has been long obſtructed, from a *Lentor*, viſcoſity, and retarded motion of the fluids in the *Uterus* and neighbouring parts, the fullneſs muſt be taken off by the abovementioned evacuations, unleſs the conſtitution be already weakened; then every thing that will gradually attenuate the fluids and quicken their circulating force, ought to be adminiſtred; ſuch as chalybeat and mercurial medicines, together with warm, bitter, and ſtomachic ingredients, aſſiſted with proper diet and exerciſe, according to the preſcriptions to be found in *Hoffman*, *Friend's Emmenologia*, and *Shaw*'s practice of phyſick.

Of

Of the FLUOR ALBUS.

The inſide membrane of the *Uterus*, according to *Aſtruc*, is thick ſet with ſmall glands, which he calls the *Colatura lactea:* Theſe, in an unimpregnated *Uterus*, ſeparate a *Mucus* that lubricates the cavity and canal of the neck, by which means the ſides are prevented from coaleſcing or growing together. The *Fluor Albus* is no other than this *Mucus* diſcharged in too great quantity; and this exceſs, when it happens from plenitude, in thoſe who feed plentifully without taking ſufficient exerciſe, is often remedied by general evacuations, ſuch as venæſection, emeticks, catharticks, and a more abſtemious diet, with a greater ſhare of exerciſe than uſual. But the cure is more difficult when the complaint is of a long ſtanding, and proceeds from a bad habit, the conſtitution being weakened by the inordinate diſcharge: In this caſe it will be neceſſary to uſe repeated emeticks, gentle exerciſe, and all thoſe medicines that contribute to ſtrengthen a lax habit of body; or if the diſtemper be cancerous, it muſt be palliated with anodynes: As to the

the form of prefcription in all thefe cafes, *Hoffman* may be confulted.

SECT. II.

Of CONCEPTION.

THE *Minutiæ*, or firft principles of bodies, being without the fphere of human comprehenfion, all that we know is by the obfervation of their effects; fo that the modus of conception is altogether uncertain, efpecially in the human fpecies, becaufe opportunities of opening pregnant women fo feldom occur.

Although the knowledge of this operation is not abfolutely neceffary for the practice of Midwifery, an inveftigation of it may not only gratify the curious, but alfo promote further enquiries; in the courfe of which many material difcoveries may be made, in the fame manner as many valuable compofitions in chymiftry were found out in the laft century, by thofe who exercifed themfelves in fearch of the philofopher's ftone.

2. From

From the time of *Hippocrates* to the ſixteenth century, it was generally believed that the *Embrio* and *Secundines* were formed by the mixture of the male and female ſemen in the *Uterus*; but during the laſt hundred years, anatomy received great improvements by the frequent diſſection of human bodies; and in ſome female ſubjects the *Fœtus* was found in one of the Fallopian tubes, in others it was diſcovered in the *Abdomen*, with the *Placenta* adhering to the ſurface of the *Viſcera*.

Malphigius and others, between the years 1650 and 1690, wrote expreſly upon the incubation of eggs, their formation, and gradual increaſe of oviparous animals: The great *Harvy* obſerved the progreſs of the viviparous kind, in a great number of different animals which he had opportunities of opening. *De Graaf* diſſected near one hundred rabbits, and is very particular and accurate in the obſervations he made. *Ruych*, *Aldes*, *Needham*, *Steno*, *Kirkringius*, *Swammerdam*, *Bartholine* the ſon, and *Drelincourt*, employed themſelves in the ſame enquiries; and in conſequence of their different remarks, a variety of theories have been erected: Yet all of them have been ſubject to many objections, and even the following, though the moſt probable, ſtill very uncertain.

When the parts in women ſubſervient to generation attain their *Acme* or full growth, one or more of the *Ova* being brought to maturity, that part of the *Peritonæum* which covers the *Ovarium* begins to ſtretch; the nervous fibres are accordingly affected, and contract themſelves ſo as to bring the *Fimbria* of the Fallopian tube in cloſe contact with the ripe *Ovum*: by which mechaniſm, this laſt is ſqueezed out of its *Nidus* or huſk, into the cavity of the tube, through which it is conveyed into the *Uterus* by a vermicular or periſtaltic motion; and if it is not immediately impregnated with an *Animalcule* of the male ſemen, muſt be diſſolved and loſt, becauſe it is now detached from the veſſels of the *Ovarium*, and has no *Vis vitæ* in itſelf.

The external coat of the *Ovum* is the membrane *Chorion*, one fourth part of which is the *Placenta*, ſuppoſed to be the root by which it was formerly joined to the veſſels

 of

of the *Ovarium*; and the navel-ſtring is no other than a continuation of the veſſels belonging to this cake.

The *Chorion* is on the inſide lined with another membrane called *Amnios*, and both are kept diſtended in a globular form, by a clear ſerous fluid, or thin *Lymph*.

As for the male ſemen, according to the obſervation of the celebrated *Lewenhoek*, it abounds with *Animalcula*, that ſwim about in it like ſo many tadpoles; and theſe are larger and more vigorous the longer the ſemen hath remained in the *Veſiculæ ſeminales*.

The parts of both male and female being thus brought to maturity, the following circumſtances are ſuppoſed to happen in coition, eſpecially in thoſe embraces which immediately follow the evacuation of the *Menſes*: In the woman, the friction of the *Penis* in the contracted *Vagina*, the repeated preſſure and ſhocks againſt the external parts, the alternate motion upwards and downwards of the *Uterus*, with its appendages the *Ovaria*, Fallopian tubes, and round ligaments, produce a general titillation and turgency; in conſequence of which the nervous fibrils are convulſed, and a fluid ejected from the proſtate or analogous glands, as well as from thoſe of the *Uterus* and Fallopian tubes: The *Fimbria* belonging to one of which, now firmly graſps the ripened *Ovum*, which at the ſame inſtant is impregnated with the male ſeed that in the orgaſm of coition had been thrown into the *Uterus*, and thence conveyed into the cavity of the tube by ſome abſorbing or convulſive power. When the two maturated principles are thus mingled, one of the *Animalcula* inſinuates itſelf into the *Ovum*, and is joined with its belly to that ruptured part of it from which the navel-ſtring is produced; or entering one of the veſſels, is protruded to the end of the *Funis*, by which a circulation is carried on from the *Embrio* to the *Placenta* and membranes. The *Ovum* being impregnated, is ſqueezed from its *Nidus* or huſk into the tube by the contraction of the *Fimbria*, and thus diſengaged from its attachments to the *Ovarium*, is endowed with a circulating force by the *Animalculum*, which has a *Vis vitæ* in itſelf: the veſſels on the ſurface of the *Ovum* being opened, in conſequence of its detachment from the *Ovarium*, abſorb the ſurrounding fluid which is ſecerned by the glands in the cavity of the tube and *Uterus*, or forced into them by motion, heat, and rarefaction, and carried along the umbilical vein, for the nouriſhment and increaſe of the impregnated maſs.

Of the ſemen that is injected or abſorbed into the *Uterus*, part is mixed with the fluid ſecreted by the glands in the canal of the neck, which is blocked up with a ſort of gluten formed by this mixture; ſo that the *Ovum* is thereby prevented from ſinking too far down, and being diſcharged.

This theory of conception, though very ingenious, and of all others the beſt ſupported with corroborating conſiderations, ſuch as, that *Fœtuſes* and *Embrios* have been actually found in the cavity of the tube, and *Abdomen*, without any marks of excluſion from the *Uterus*; beſides other preſumptions that will be mentioned when we come to treat of the nutrition of the *Fœtus*; I ſay, notwithſtanding the plauſibility of the ſcheme, it is attended with circumſtances which are hitherto inexplicable; namely, the

the manner in which the *Animalculum* gains admiſſion into the *Ovum*, either while it remains in the *Ovarium*, ſojourns in the tube, or is depoſited in the *Fundus Uteri*; and the method by which the veſſels of the navel-ſtring are inoſculated with thoſe of the *Animalculum*. Indeed, theſe points are ſo intricate, that every different theoriſt has ſtarted different opinions concerning them, ſome of which are rather jocular than inſtructive.

SECT. III.

Of the increaſe of the UTERUS *after conception.*

IT is ſuppoſed, that the *Ovum* ſwims in a fluid, which it abſorbs ſo as to increaſe gradually in magnitude, 'till it comes in contact with all the inner ſurface of the *Fundus*; and this being diſtended in proportion to the augmentation of its contents, the upper part of the neck begins alſo to be ſtretched.

About the third month of geſtation, the *Ovum* in bigneſs equals a gooſe egg; and then, nearly one fourth of the neck at its upper part, is diſtended equal with the *Fundus*. At the fifth month, the *Fundus* is increaſed to a much greater magnitude, and rises upwards to the middle space betwixt the upper part of the *Pubis* and the navel, and at that period, one half of the neck is extended. At seven months, the *Fundus* reaches as high as the navel: at the eighth month, it is advanced midway between the navel and *Scrobiculum cordis*; and in the ninth month is raised quite up to this last mentioned part, the neck of the womb being then altogether distended.

Now that the whole substance of the *Uterus* is stretched, the neck and *Os Internum*, which were at first the strongest, become the weakest parts of the womb, and the stretching force being still continued by the increase of the *Fœtus* and secundines, which are extended by the inclosed waters in a globular form, the *Os Uteri* begins gradually to give way. In the beginning of its dilatation, the nervous fibres in this place being more sensible than any other part of the *Uterus*, are irritated and, yield an uneasy sensation; to alleviate which, the woman squeezes her *Uterus*, by contracting the abdominal muscles, and at the same time filling the lungs with air, by which the *Diaphragm* is

kept

kept down; the pain being rather increaſed than abated by this ſtraining, is communicated to all the neighbouring parts, to which the ligaments and veſſels are attached; ſuch as the back, loins, and inſide of the thighs; and by this compreſſion of the *Uterus*, the waters and membranes are ſqueezed againſt the *Os Uteri*, which is of conſequence a little more opened.

The woman being unable to continue this effort, for any length of time, from the violence of the pain it occaſions, and the ſtrength of the muſcles being thereby a little exhauſted and impaired; the contracting force abates, the tenſion of the *Os Tincæ* being taken off, it becomes more ſoft, and contracts a little; ſo that the nervous fibres are relaxed. This remiſſion of pain the patient enjoys for ſome time, until the ſame increaſing force renews the ſtretching pains, irritation, and ſomething like a teneſmus at the *Os Uteri*; the compreſſion of the womb again takes place, and the internal mouth is a little more dilated, either by the preſſure of the waters and membranes, or when the fluid is in ſmall quantity, by the child's head forced down by the contraction of the *Uterus*,

rus, which in that caſe is in contact with the body of the *Fœtus.*

In this manner the labour pains begin and continue to return periodically, growing ſtronger and more frequent, until the *Os Uteri* is fully dilated, the membranes are depreſſed and broke; ſo that the waters are diſcharged, the *Uterus* contracts, and with the aſſiſtance of the muſcles, the child is forced along and delivered.

Although this account may be liable to objections, eſpecially in thoſe caſes when the child is delivered before the full time; it neverthelefs ſeems more probable than that hypotheſis, which imputes the labour pains, to the motion of the child calcitrating the *Uterus*: for, it frequently happens, that the woman never feels the child ſtir during the whole time of labour, and dead children are delivered as eaſily as thoſe that come alive, except when the birth is retarded by the body's being ſwelled to an extraordinary ſize.

SECT.

SECT. IV.

Of the magnitude, weight, and different appellations given to the Ovum *and* Child.

WHEN the *Ovum* deſcends into the *Uterus*, it is ſuppoſed to be about the ſize of a poppy-ſeed, and in the third month, augmented to the bigneſs of a gooſe egg. Ten days after conception, the child (according to ſome authors) weighs half a grain, at thirty days, is increaſed to the weight of twenty two grains, at three months, weighs betwixt two and three ounces; and at nine months, from ten to twelve, and ſometimes ſixteen pounds: by which calculation it would appear, that the progreſs of the *Fœtus* is quickeſt in the beginning of its growth: for, from the tenth to the thirtieth day, (according to this ſuppoſition) it increaſes to three and forty times its weight. All theſe calculations are uncertain.

The conception is called an *Embrio*, until all the parts are diſtinctly formed, generally in the third month, and from that period to delivery, is diſtinguiſhed by the appellation of *Fœtus*.

SECT. V.

Of Twins.

WHEN two or more children are included in the *Uterus*, at the ſame time, each has a ſeparate *Placenta*, with umbilical cords and veſſels: ſometimes theſe *Placent* are altogether diſtinct, and at other times they form but one cake.

Yet, by an inſtance that lately fell under my obſervation, it appears, that ſometimes twins have but one *Placenta* in common: whether or not there were two ſets of membranes, I could not diſcover, becauſe they had been tore off by the gentleman who delivered the woman; but, when the artery in one of the navel-ſtrings was injected, the matter flowed out at one of the veſſels belonging to the other, and the communication between them is ſtill viſible, though they are ſeparated at the diſtance of three or four inches.

When two children are diſtinct, they are called twins; and monſters when they are joined together; the firſt (according to the foregoing theory) are produced when different

ent *Animalcula* impregnate different *Ova*; and the laſt are engendered when two or more *Animalcula* introduce themſelves, and are included in one *Ovum*.

SECT. VI.

Of SUPERFOETATION.

IT was formerly imagined that a woman might conceive a ſecond time during pregnancy, and be delivered of one child, ſome weeks or months before the other could be ready for the world: but this opinion is now excluded by ſome; becauſe, the *Ovum* fills the whole *Fundus Uteri*, and the gelatinous ſubſtance already mentioned, locks up the neck and *Os Internum*, ſo as to hinder more ſemen from entering the womb and impregnating a ſecond egg, in any ſubſequent coition. Wherefore, in all thoſe caſes which gave riſe to this ſuppoſition, it may be taken for granted, that the woman was actually with child of twins, one of which, lying near the *Os Internum*, might chance to die and mortify, ſo as that the membranes give way, and the dead *Fœtus* is diſcharged, while the other remains in the *Uterus*,

Uterus, and is delivered at the full time. On the other hand, by ſome accident, the firſt and largeſt may be born ſome days or weeks before the full time, and afterwards the *Os Tincæ* contracts ſo as to detain the other 'till the due period. At other times, the child that lies next to the *Fundus*, is the ſmalleſt, and follows after the birth of the other, ſometimes dead and putrified, and ſometimes in an emaciated condition.

SECT. VII.

Of ABORTIONS.

A Miſcarriage that happens before the tenth day, was formerly called an efflux, becauſe the *Embrio* and ſecundines are not then formed, and nothing but the liquid conception, or *Genitura* is diſcharged. From the tenth day to the third month, it was known by the term expulſion, the *Embrio* and ſecundines being ſtill ſo ſmall, that the woman is in no great danger from violent flooding.

If ſhe parted with her burthen betwixt that period and the ſeventh month, ſhe was ſaid to ſuffer an abortion; in which caſe ſhe underwent

underwent greater danger, and was deliver-ed with more difficulty than before; becauſe the *Uterus* and veſſels being more diſtended, a larger quantity of blood was loſt in a ſhorter time, the *Fœtus* was increaſed in bulk, and the neck of the womb not yet fully ſtretch-ed; beſides, ſhould the child be born alive, it will be ſo ſmall and tender that it will not ſuck, and ſcarce receive any ſort of nouriſh-ment.

When delivery happens between the ſe-venth month and full time, the woman is ſaid to be in labour: but, inſtead of theſe diſtinctions, if ſhe loſes her burden at any time from conception to the ſeventh or eighth, or even in the ninth month, we now ſay indiſcriminately, ſhe has miſcarried, or parted with child.

Hippocrates alledges, that a child born in the ſeventh month, ſometimes lives; where-as, if it comes in the eighth, it will proba-bly die, becauſe all healthy children (ſays he) make an effort to be delivered in the ſeventh month, and if they are not then born, and the *Niſus* is repeated in the eighth, when the child muſt be weakened by its former un-

ſucceſsful

ſucceſsful attempt, and therefore not likely to live; whereas, ſhould the ſecond effort be deferred 'till the ninth, the *Fœtus* will, by that time, be ſufficiently recovered from the fatigue it had undergone in the ſeventh. Experience, however, contradicts this aſſertion; for the older the child is, we find it always (*cæteris paribus*) the ſtronger, conſequently the more hardy and eaſily nurſed: neither is there any ſufficient reaſon for adhering to the opinion of *Pythagoras* on this ſubject, who declares that number eight is not ſo fortunate as ſeven or nine.

The common term of pregnancy is limited to nine ſolar months, reckoning from the laſt diſcharge of the *Catamenia*: yet in ſome, tho' very few, uterine geſtation exceeds that period; and as this is a poſſible caſe, we ought always to judge on the charitable ſide, in the perſuaſion, that it is better ſeveral guilty perſons ſhould eſcape, than one innocent woman ſuffer in point of reputation.

SECT. VIII.

Of false CONCEPTIONS *and* MOLES.

IT was formerly ſuppoſed, that if the parts of the *Embrio* and ſecundines were not ſeparated and diſtinctly formed from the mixture of the male and female ſemen, they formed a maſs, which when diſcharged before the fourth month, was called a falſe conception; if it continued longer in the *Uterus*, ſo as to increaſe in magnitude, it went under the denomination of a *Mola*. But theſe things are now to be accounted for, in a more probable and certain manner. Should the *Embrio* die (ſuppoſe in the firſt or ſecond month) ſome days before it is diſcharged, it will ſometimes be intirely diſſolved, ſo that when the ſecundines are delivered, there is nothing elſe to be ſeen. In the firſt month the *Embrio* is ſo ſmall and tender, that this diſſolution will be performed in twelve hours; in the ſecond month, two, three, or four days will ſuffice for this purpoſe; and even in the third month, it will be diſſolved in fourteen or fifteen: beſides, the blood frequently forms thick *Lamina*

mina round the *Ovum*, to the ſurface of which they adhere ſo ſtrongly, that it is very difficult to diſtinguiſh what part is *Placenta*, and what membrane. Even after the *Embrio* and *Placenta* are diſcharged, in the ſecond or third month, the mouth and neck of the womb are often ſo cloſely contracted, that the fibrous part of the blood is retained in the *Fundus*, ſometimes to the fifth or ſeventh day; and when it comes off, exhibits the appearance of an *Ovum*, the external ſurface, by the ſtrong preſſure of the *Uterus*, reſembling a membrane; ſo that the whole is miſtaken for a falſe conception.

This ſubſtance, in bigneſs, commonly equals a pigeon or hen egg; or if it exceeds that ſize, and is longer retained, is diſtinguiſhed by the apellation of *Mola*: but this laſt generally happens in women betwixt the age of forty five and fifty, or later, when their *Menſes* begin to diſappear; ſometimes from internal or external accidents that may produce continued floodings. If the *Catamenia* have ceaſed to flow for ſome time, in elderly women, and return with pain, ſuch a ſymptom is frequently the fore-runner of a cancer;

cancer; before or after this happens, ſometimes a large fleſh-like ſubſtance will be diſcharged with great pain, reſembling that of labour; and upon examination, appears to be no more than the fibrous part of the blood, which aſſumes that form by being long preſſed in the *Uterus* or *Vagina*.

In this place, it will not be amiſs to obſerve, that the glands of the *Uterus* and *Vagina* will ſometimes increaſe, and diſtend the adjacent parts to a ſurpriſing degree: if (for example) one of the glands of the *Uterus* be ſo obſtructed as that there is a preſſure on the returning vein and excretory duct, the arterial blood will gradually ſtretch the ſmaller veſſels, and conſequently increaſe the ſize of the gland, which will grow larger and larger, as long as the force of the impelled fluid is greater than the reſiſtance of the veſſels that contain it; by which means, a very ſmall gland will be inlarged to a great bulk, and the *Uterus* gradually ſtretched as in uterine geſtation, though the progreſs may be ſo ſlow as to be protracted for years inſtead of months. Nevertheleſs, the *Os Internum* will be dilated, and the gland (if not too large to paſs) will be ſqueezed into the *Vagina*, provided it adheres to the *Uterus*, by a ſmall neck; nay, it will lengthen more and more, ſo as to appear on the outſide of the *Os Externum*; in which caſe it may be eaſily ſeparated by a ligature. This diſeaſe will be the ſooner known and eaſier remedied, the lower its origin in the *Uterus* is. But ſhould the gland take its riſe in the *Vagina*, hard by the mouth of the womb, it will ſhew itſelf ſtill ſooner, and a ligature may be eaſily introduced, provided the tumour is not ſo large as to fill up the cavity, and hinder the neck of it from being commodiouſly felt. Though the greateſt difficulty occurs when the gland is confined to the *Uterus*, being too much enlarged to paſs through the *Os Internum*.

Sometimes all or moſt of the glands in the *Uterus* are thus affected, and augment the womb to ſuch a degree, that it will weigh a great many pounds, and the woman is deſtroyed by its preſſure upon the ſurrounding parts: but ſhould this indolent ſtate of the tumour be altered by any accident that will produce irritation and inflammation,

mation, the parts will grow ſchirrous, and a cancer enſue.

This misfortune, for the moſt part, happens to women when their menſtrual evacuations leave them ; and ſometimes (though ſeldom) to child-bearing women, in conſequence of ſevere labour.

Some people have affirmed, that the *Placenta* being left in the *Uterus*, after the delivery of the child, grows gradually larger: but the contrary of this aſſertion is proved by common practice, from which it appears, that the *Placenta* is actually preſſed into ſmaller dimenſions, and ſometimes into a ſubſtance almoſt demi-cartilaginous : for, after the death or delivery of the child, the ſecundines receive no farther increaſe or growth. Dropſies and hydatids are alſo ſuppoſed to be formed in the *Uterus*, and diſcharged from thence, together with air or wind : the *Ovaria* are ſometimes affected in the ſame manner, are inflamed, impoſtumate, grow ſchirrous, cancerous, and the patient is deſtroyed by the diſcharge, which gradually fi ls the *Abdomen* with *Pus* and *Ichor* ; ſo that all theſe complaints, if known, ought to be obviated in the beginning.

SECT. IX.

Of the PLACENTA.

I Have already obſerved, that the *Ovum* is formed of the *Placenta*, with the *Chorion* and *Amnios*, which are globularly diſtended by the incloſed waters that ſurround the child. The *Placenta* is commonly of a round figure, ſomewhat reſembling an oat-cake, about ſix inches in diameter, and one inch thick in the middle, growing a little thinner towards the circumference: it is compoſed of veins and arteries, which are divided into an infinite number of ſmall branches, the venous part of which unite in one large tube, called the umbilical vein, which brings back the blood, and is ſuppoſed to carry along the nutritive fluid from the veſſels of the *Chorion* and *Placenta* to the child, whoſe belly it perforates at the navel; from thence paſſing into the liver, where it communicates with the *Vena Portarum* and *Cava*. It is furniſhed with two arteries, which ariſe from the inter-

nal

nal *Iliacs* of the child, and running up on each ſide of the bladder, perforate the belly where the umbilical vein entered; then they proceed to the *Placenta* in a ſpiral line, twining around the vein, in conjunction with which, they form the *Funiculus Umbilicalis*, which is commonly four or five hand-breadths in length; ſometimes only two or three, and ſometimes it extends to the length of eight or ten. The two arteries, on their arrival at the inner ſurface of the *Placenta*, are divided and ſubdivided into minute branches, which at laſt end in ſmall capillaries that inoſculate with the veins of the ſame order. Theſe arteries, together with the umbilical vein, are ſuppoſed to do the ſame office in the *Placenta* which is afterwards performed in the lungs by the pulmonary artery and vein, until the child is delivered and begins to breathe: and this opinion ſeems to be confirmed by the following experiments. If the child and *Placenta* are both delivered ſuddenly, or the laſt immediately after the firſt, and if the child, though alive, does not yet breathe, the blood may be felt circulating, ſometimes ſlowly, at other times, with great force through the arteries of the *Funis*, to the *Placenta*, and from thence back again to the child along the umbilical vein. When the veſſels are ſlightly preſſed, the arteries ſwell between the preſſure and the child, while the vein grows turgid between that and the *Placenta*; from the ſurface of which no blood is obſerved to flow, although it be lying in a baſin, among warm water. As the child begins to breathe, the circulation, though it was weak before, immediately grows ſtronger and ſtronger, and then in a few minutes the pulſation in the navel-ſtring becomes more languid, and at laſt intirely ſtops. If, after the child is delivered, and the navel-ſtring cut, provided the *Placenta* adheres firmly to the *Uterus*, which is thereby kept extended; or if the womb is ſtill diſtended by another child, no more blood flows from the umbilical veſſels, than what ſeemed to be contained in them at the inſtant of cutting; and this, in common caſes, does not exceed the quantity of two or three ounces: and finally, when in conſequence of violent floodings, the mother expires, either in time of deli-

very,

very, or ſoon after it, the child is ſometimes found alive and vigorous.

The external ſurface of the *Placenta* is divided into ſeveral lobes, that it may yield and conform itſelf more commodiouſly with the inner ſurface of the *Uterus* to which it adheres, ſo as to prevent its being ſeparated by any ſhock or blows upon the *Abdomen*, unleſs when violent.

Thoſe groupes of veins and arteries which enter into the compoſition of the *Placenta*, receive external coats from the *Chorion*, which is the outward membrane of the *Ovum*, thick and ſtrong, and forms three fourths of the external globe that contains the waters and the child; the remaining part being covered by the *Placenta*; ſo that theſe two in conjunction conſtitute the whole external ſurface of the *Ovum*. Some indeed, alledge, that theſe are inveloped with a cribriform or cellular ſubſtance, by which they ſeem to adhere by contact only to the *Uterus*; and that the inner membrane of the womb is full of little glands, whoſe excretory ducts opening into the *Fundus* and neck, ſecrete a ſoft, thin mucus (as formerly obſerved) to lubricate the whole cavity of the *Uterus*, which beginning to ſtretch in time of geſtation, the veſſels that compoſe theſe glands are alſo diſtended, conſequently a greater quantity of this mucus is ſeparated and retained in this ſuppoſed cribriform and cellular ſubſtance, the abſorbing veſſels of which take it in, and convey it along the veins, for the nouriſhment of the child. The womb being therefore diſtended in proportion to the increaſe of the child, thoſe glands are alſo proportionably enlarged; by which means a larger quantity of the fluid is ſeparated, becauſe the nutriment of the child muſt be augmented in proportion to the progreſs of its growth: and this liquor undergoes an alteration in quality as well as in quantity, being changed from a clear, thin fluid, into the more viſcous conſiſtence of milk. In ſome caſes this mucus hath been diſcharged from the *Uterus*, in time of pregnancy, and both mother and child weakened by the evacuation, which may be occaſioned by the *Chorion*'s adhering too looſely, or being in one part actually ſeparated from the womb.

Formerly, it was taken for granted by many, that the *Placenta* always adhered to the

the *Fundus Uteri*; but this notion is refuted by certain obſervations, in conſequence of which, we find it as often ſticking to the ſides, back, and foreparts, and ſometimes, as far down as the inſide of the *Os Uteri*.

When the *Placenta* is delivered, and no other part of the membrane tore except that through which the child paſſed, the opening is generally near the edge or ſide of the *Placenta*, and ſeldom in the middle of the membranes; and a hog's bladder being introduced at this opening, and inflated, when laying in water, will ſhew the ſhape and ſize of the inner ſurface of the womb, and plainly diſcover the part to which the *Placenta* adhered.

The *Chorion* is on the inſide lined with the *Amnios*, which is a thin, tranſparent membrane, without any veſſels ſo large as to admit the red globules of blood: it adheres to the *Chorion* by contact, and ſeems to form the external coat of the *Funis Umbilicalis*.

This membrane contains the *Serum* in which the child ſwims, which fluid is ſuppoſed to be furniſhed by lymphatic veſſels that open into the inner ſurface of the *Amnios*.

nios. If this liquid is neither abſorbed into the body of the *Fœtus*, or taken into the ſtomach, by ſuction at the mouth, there muſt be abſorbing veſſels in this membrane, in the ſame manner as in the *Abdomen* and other cavities of the body, where there is a conſtant renovation of humidity.

The quantity of this fluid, in proportion to the weight of the *Fœtus*, is much greater in the firſt than in the laſt month of geſtation, being in the one perhaps ten times the weight of the *Embrio* ; whereas in the other, it is commonly in the proportion of one to two : for ſix pounds of water ſurrounding a *Fœtus* that weighs twelve pound, is reckoned a large proportion, the quantity being often much leſs ; nay, ſometimes there is very little or none at all.

In moſt animals of the brute ſpecies, there is a third membrane called *Allantois*, which reſembles a long and wide blind gut, and contains the urine of the *Fœtus* : it is ſituated between the *Chorion* and *Amnios*, and commmunicates with the *Urachus* that riſes from the *Fundus* of the bladder, and runs along with the umbilical veſſels, depoſiting the

the urine in this reſervoir, which is attached to its other extremity. This bag hath not yet been certainly diſcovered in the human *Fœtus*, the *Urachus* of which, though plainly perceivable, ſeems hitherto, to be quite imperforated.

From the foregoing obſervations upon nutrition, it ſeems probable, that the *Fœtus* is rather nouriſhed by the abſorption of the nutritive fluid into the veſſels of the *Placenta* and *Chorion*, than from the red blood circulated in full ſtream from the arteries of the *Uterus* to the veins of the *Placenta*, and returned by the arteries of the laſt to the veins of the firſt, in order to be renewed, refined, and made arterial blood in the lungs of the mother.

Yet this doctrine of abſorption, is clogged with one objection, which hath never been fully anſwered; namely, that if the *Placenta* adheres to the lower part of the *Uterus*, when the *Os Internum* begins to be dilated, a flooding immediately enſues; and the ſame ſymptom happens upon a partial or total ſeparation of the *Placenta* from any other part of the womb; whereas no ſuch conſequence follows a ſeparation of the *Chorion*.

The

The new theorifts indeed, obferve, that there is no neceffity for a fupply of red blood from the mother; becaufe the circulating force in the veffels of the *Fœtus*, produces heat and motion fufficient to endue the fluids with a fanguine colour; that neither is there occafion for returning and refining this blood in the lungs of the mother, becaufe that office is fufficiently performed in the *Placenta*, until the *Fœtus* is delivered, when its own lungs are put to their proper ufe; and laftly, that the blood of the mother is too grofs a fluid to anfwer the occafions of the *Fœtus*. Certain it is, the chick in the egg, is nourifhed by the white which is forced along the veffels, and the quantity of red blood increafes in proportion to the growth of the contained *Embrio* or *Fœtus*, without any fupply from the hen.

On the whole, the opinions broached upon the nutrition of the *Embrio* and *Fœtus* in *Utero*, have been as various as thofe that are adopted concerning the modus of conception.

BOOK

BOOK II.

CHAP. I.

Of the diseases incident to pregnant women, being either such as immediately proceed from pregnancy, or such as may happen at any other time, and if not carefully prevented or removed, may be of dangerous consequence both to mother and child.

SECT. I.

Of NAUSEA *and* VOMITING.

THE first complaint attending pregnancy, is the nausea and vomiting, which in some women begins soon after conception, and frequently continues 'till the end of the fourth month. Most women are troubled with this symptom, more or less, particularly vomitings in the morning:

morning: ſome who have no ſuch complaint in one pregnancy ſhall be violently attacked with it in another; and in a few, it prevails during the whole time of uterine geſtation.

The vomiting (if not very violent) is ſeldom of dangerous conſequence; but on the contrary, is ſuppoſed to be ſerviceable to the patient, by unloading the ſtomach of ſuperfluous nouriſhment, thereby carrying off or preventing too great a turgency in the veſſels of the *Viſcera* and *Uterus*; and by creating a kind of needing motion, which will aſſiſt the *Fundus* and neck of the womb in ſtretching. Neverthleſs, if the ſtraining is too great, it may endanger a miſcarriage.

Perhaps this complaint is chiefly occaſioned by a fullneſs of the veſſels of the *Uterus*, owing to the obſtructed *Catamenia*, the whole quantity of which, cannot as yet be employed in the nutrition of the *Embrio*: over and above this cauſe, it has been ſuppoſed that the *Uterus* being ſtretched by the increaſe of the *Ovum*, a tenſion of the parts enſues, affecting the nerves of that *Viſcus*; eſpecially thoſe that ariſe from the *Sympathetici Maximi*, and communicate with the *Plexus*, at the mouth of the ſtomach. Whatever

ever be the caufe, the complaint is beft relieved by blooding, more or lefs, acording to the *Plethora* and ftrength of the patient, and if fhe is coftive, by emollient glyfters and opening medicines, that will evacuate the hardened contents of the *Colon* and *Rectum*; fo that the *Vifcera* will be rendered light and eafy, and the ftretching fullnefs of the veffels taken off. A light, nutritive and fpare diet, with moderate exercife, and a free open air, will conduce to the removal of this complaint.

SECT. II.

Of difficulty in making water, coftivenefs, fwelling of the Hœmorrhoids, *legs, and* Labia Pudendi; *and the* Dyfpnœa *and vomiting at the latter end of pregnancy.*

TOWARDS the end of the fourth month, or beginning of the fifth, the *Uterus* is fo much diftended as to fill all the upper part of the *Pelvis*, and then it begins to rife upwards into the *Abdomen*: about the fame time the *Os Internum* is likewife raifed and turned backwards towards the *Sacrum*, becaufe the *Fundus* is inclined forwards in its rife. The *Uterus*, according to the different directions in which it distends, produces various complaints by its weight and pressure upon the adjacent parts, whether in the *Pelvis*, or higher on the *Abdomen*. In the fourth or fifth month, it presses against the *Sphincter* of the bladder in the *Pelvis*, and produces a difficulty in making water, and sometimes (though seldom) a total suppression. This complaint will happen, if the womb is sunk too low in the *Vagina*, or if the *Ovum*, instead of adhering to the *Fundus*, descends into the wide part in the middle of the neck, which accordingly first undergoes distension. This disposition of the *Ovum* is frequently the cause of abortion, because the mouth and neck being in this case, from the stretching, the weakest parts of the *Uterus*, the *Os Internum* begins to be opened too soon: yet sometimes, this will continue strong and rigid, and after the neck is enlarged, the *Fundus* will be last of all stretched till the end of gestation, and the woman be happily delivered *.

* This is one probable reason to account for the *Placenta's* sometimes adhering over the inside of the mouth of the womb, and helps to support the theory of the neck's turning shorter and shorter, as the full time approaches.

But,

But, as the ſtretching begins lower down in this, than in a common caſe, the *Uterus* muſt conſequently preſs againſt all parts of the *Pelvis*, before it can riſe above the brim; and this preſſure ſometimes produces an obſtruction of urine, and difficulty in going to ſtool: the general compreſſion of all theſe parts will be attended with a degree of inflammation in the ſubſtance of the *Uterus*, the *Vagina*, mouth of the bladder and *Rectum*; from whence violent pains and a fever will enſue. In order to remove or alleviate theſe ſymptoms, recourſe muſt be had to bleeding and glyſters, the urine muſt be drawn off by the catheter, fomentations and warm baths be uſed, and this method occaſionally repeated until the complaints abate; and they commonly vaniſh in conſequence of the womb's riſing higher, ſo as to be ſupported on the brim of the *Pelvis*.

By the preſſure of the *Uterus* upon the upper part of the *Rectum* and lower part of the *Colon*, where it makes ſemicircular turns to the right and left, the *Fæces* are hindered to paſs, and by remaining too long in the guts, are indurated, the fluid parts being abſorbed by the lacteal veſſels: hence ariſes violent ſtraining at ſtool, and a compreſſion of the womb, which threatens abortion. When the patient, therefore, has laboured under this ſymptom for ſeveral days, let emollient, laxative, and gently ſtimulating glyſters be injected: but if the *Rectum* be ſo obſtructed as that the injection cannot paſs, ſuppoſitories are firſt to be introduced; for, frequently, when the *Colon* and *Rectum* are compreſſed by the *Uterus*, the periſtaltic motion is weakened and impeded, ſo that the guts cannot expel their contents; in which caſe the ſuppoſitory by irritation quickens this faculty, and in diſſolving, lubricates the parts, thereby facilitating the diſcharge of the hardened *Fæces*. This previous meaſure being taken, a glyſter ought to be injected, in order to diſſolve the collected and indurated contents of the *Colon*, as well as to lubricate and ſtimulate the inſide of that inteſtine, ſo as to effect a general evacuation; and for this purpoſe, a ſyringe ſhould be uſed inſtead of a bladder, that the injection may be thrown up with greater efficacy and force.

Theſe glyſters ought to be repeated until the hardened *Fæces* are altogether brought away,

away, and the laſt diſcharge appears to be of a ſoft conſiſtence: neither ought the preſcriber to truſt to the reports of the patient or nurſe, but to his own ſenſes in examining the effects of theſe injections; for if the complaint hath continued ſeveral days, a large quantity of indurated *Fæces* ought to be diſcharged. To avoid ſuch inconvenience for the future, an emollient glyſter muſt be injected every ſecond night; or if the patient will not ſubmit to this method, which is certainly the eaſieſt and beſt, recourſe muſt be had to thoſe lenients mentioned at the latter end of this ſection; for when the *Fæces* are long retained, the air rarifies, expands, and ſtretches the *Colon*, producing ſevere cholic pains; this being the method followed by nature, with a view to diſburthen herſelf when ſhe is thus encumbered.

The preſſure of the *Uterus* upon the hæmorrhoidal and internal *Iliac* veins, produces a turgency and tumefaction of all the parts below, ſuch as the *Pudenda*, *Vagina*, *Anus*, and even the *Os internum*, and neck of the womb. This tumefaction of the hæmorrhoidal veins, appears in those swellings at the inside and outside of the *Anus*, which are known by the name of the external and internal *Hæmorrhoids*, or piles. This is a complaint to which women are naturally more subject than is the other sex; but it is always most violent in time of pregnancy, when the same method of cure may be administred as that practised at other times, though greater caution must be used in applying leeches to the parts; because, in this case, a great quantity of blood may be lost before the discharge can be restrained.

About the latter end of the fifth, or in the beginning of the sixth month, the *Uterus* being stretched above the brim, and the *Fundus* raised to the middle space betwixt the *Pubis* and navel, is considerably increased in weight; and even then (though much more so near the full time) lies heavy upon the upper part of the brim, presses upon the *Vertebræ* of the loins and *Ossa ilia*, and rising still higher with an augmented force, gradually stretches the *Parietes* of the *Abdomen*, pushing the intestines upwards and to each side.

The

The weight and preſſure of the external *Iliac* veins, is attended with a ſurcharge or fullneſs in the returning veſſels that come from the feet, legs, and thighs; and this tumefaction produces œdematous and inflammatory ſwellings in theſe parts, together with varicus tumours in the veins, that ſometimes come to ſuppuration.

The ſame weight and preſſure occaſion pains in the back, belly, and loins, eſpecially towards the end of the eighth, or in the ninth month: if the *Uterus* riſes too high, a *Dyſpnæa* or difficulty in breathing, and frequent vomitings enſue; the firſt proceeds from the confinement of the lungs and *Diaphragm* in reſpiration, the liver and *Viſcera* of the *Abdomen* being forced up into the *Thorax*; and the laſt is occaſioned by the extraordinary preſſure upon the ſtomach.

All the complaints above deſcribed; namely, ſwelling of the legs, thighs, and *Labia pudendi*, pains in the back, loins, and belly, with *Dyſpnæa* and vomiting, are removed or palliated by the following method: The patient (if ſhe can bear ſuch evacuations) is generally relieved by bleeding at the arm or ancle, to the amount of eight or ten ounces; but the quantity muſt be proportioned to the emergency of the caſe: the belly muſt be kept open and eaſy with emollient glyſters and laxative medicines, ſuch as a ſpoonful or two of a mixture compoſed of equal parts of *Ol. Amygd. d.* and *Syr. Violar.* taken every night; or from two drachms to half an ounce of manna, or the ſame quantity of lenitive electuary; a ſmall doſe of rhubarb, or five grains of any opening pill, unleſs the patient be troubled with the *Hæmorrhoids*, in which caſe all aloetic medicines ought to be avoided: the patient muſt not walk much, or undergo hard exerciſe, but frequently reſt upon the bed, and lie longer than uſual in the morning. When the ſwelling of the legs is moderate, and only returns at night, rollers or the laced ſtocking may be ſerviceable; but when it extends in a great degree to the thighs, *Labia pudendi*, and lower part of the belly, in a woman of a full habit of body, venæſection is neceſſary, becauſe this œdematous ſwelling proceeds from a compreſſion of the returning veins, and not from laxity, as in the *Anaſarca* and leucophlegmatick conſtitutions; here

here moderate exerciſe, and (as I have already obſerved) frequent reſting on a bed or couch, is beneficial; or if the ſkin of the legs and *Pudenda* is exceſſively ſtretched, ſo as to be violently pained, the patient will be greatly relieved by punćturing the parts occaſionally: but theſe complaints cannot be totally removed till delivery, after which they commonly vaniſh of themſelves.

The bellies of thoſe that are indolent and uſe no exerciſe, ought to be moderately compreſſed, ſo that the *Uterus* may not riſe too high, and occaſion difficulty in breathing, and vomiting, in the laſt months; but they muſt not be too ſtraitly ſwathed, leſt the womb ſhould be determined, in ſtretching, over the *Pubis*, and produce a pendulous belly, which is often the cauſe of difficult labours. A medium ought therefore to be preſerved in this article of compreſſing, and no woman lace her jumps or ſtays ſo as to make herſelf uneaſy: while the diet, air, and exerciſe, ought to be regulated according to the conſtitution, cuſtom, and complaints of the patient.

CHAP. II.

Of the Diseases incident to pregnant Women.

SECT. I.

Of the STONE *in the* KIDNEYS *and* BLADDER.

WOMEN are frequently afflicted with small stones and gravel in the kidneys, being less subject than men to this complaint in the bladder, because their *Urethras* are short and wide, and suffer the calculous concretions to pass with the urine more easily.

In pregnancy, it is often difficult to distinguish gravelly pains from those that are felt in the small of the back and loins, proceeding from the pressure of the *Uterus* upon these parts: in both cases, when the pains are violent, the urine is high coloured, and the difference is, that in the gravel a quantity of sand generally falls to the bottom; though the sediment commonly deposited by high coloured urine is often mistaken for gravel:

gravel: this miſtake, however, is the leſs material, becauſe both complaints is relieved by the ſame method, namely, venæſection, emollient glyſters, emulſions, with gum arabic, infuſions of *Althea*, *Sem. Lini* and *Opiates*, and an application of *Emplaſt. Roborans* to the back.

Pains in the loins and belly, extending to the falſe ribs, occaſioned by the ſtretching of the *Uterus*, are eaſed by rubbing and anointing the parts every night before the fire with emollient unguents, ſuch as that of *Althea*, *&c.*

In pregnant women, the complaints from a ſtone in the bladder (which is ſometimes, though ſeldom, the caſe) are to be treated in the ſame manner as at any other time; except that when the patient is near delivery, it is not adviſeable to endeavour to extract it, leſt the operation ſhould be attended with an inflammation of the *Urethra* and *Vagina*: if therefore the ſtone ſhould be rough, angular, or ſurrounded with ſharp prickles, the woman ſuffers greatly from the preſſure of the *Uterus* upon the bladder, eſpecially in time of labour, when the membranes are broke,

broke, and the head of the child is pushed into the upper part of the *Pelvis*; because the stone is then pressed before it upon the neck of the bladder, so as to occasion exquisite torture, and infallibly retard the labour-pains. If the stone hath descended into the *Meatus urinarius*, perhaps it may be easily extracted; but if it still remains within the bladder, the only way of relieving the patient is by introducing a *Catheter*, also one or two fingers into the *Vagina*, to push up the stone above and behind the head of the child; or if this cannot be done, to turn and deliver by the feet, before the head is pressed too far down in the *Pelvis*.

SECT. II.

Of HERNIAS, *or* RUPTURES.

WOMEN are also afflicted with ruptures in different parts, such as the navel, groin, and *Pelvis*; but as the *Uterus* in time of gestation stretches higher and higher, the *Omentum* and intestines are pressed more and more upward and to each side; and about the fifth or sixth month, the womb riſes ſo high, that the inteſtine cannot deſcend into the groin, and the rupture in that part ceaſes for the preſent. About the eighth month, the *Uterus* is ſo high advanced, that the inteſtine or *Epiplon* is kept from puſhing out at the navel, conſequently the umbilcial *Hernia* is likewiſe ſuſpended till after delivery; but this will not happen in either caſe, unleſs the rupture be of that kind that ſuffers the *Omentum* and inteſtine to be eaſily reduced.

Women are chiefly ſubject to ruptures of the *Umbilicus*, and thoſe of the groin moſt incident to the other ſex; but there is a third kind peculiar to women, though it rarely happens even in them: this is produced from the inteſtine falling down betwixt the back-part of the *Uterus* and *Vagina*, and the fore-part of the *Rectum*. The *Peritoneum* deſcends much lower in this place than at the anterior deſcent, where it covers the upper part of the bladder, or at the ſides of the *Pelvis*, where it forms the *Ligamenta lata*; for it reaches to within one or two inches of the *Perineum*, and the inteſtines preſſing it farther down, or burſting it in

this

this part, are puſhed out in the form of a large tumour, at the ſide of the *Perineum*, betwixt the lower part of the *Iſchium* and *Coccyx*. The gut being ſo ſituated in time of labour, when the child's head is ſqueezed into the *Pelvis*, may ſuffer ſtrangulation if the caſe ſhould prove lingering and tedious, and the preſſure continue for any length of time. In order to prevent or remedy this accident, let the *Os externum* be gradualiy opened with the hand, which being introduced in the *Vagina*, ſhall raiſe the child's head, ſo as to ſuffer the inteſtine to be puſhed above it by the aſſiſtance of the other hand, which preſſes upon the outſide: in this manner both hands may be uſed alternately, till the purpoſe be effected; or ſhould this method fail to reduce and retain the inteſtine, the child muſt be delivered with the forceps, or turned and brought by the feet, as we have directed in the caſe of a ſtone in the bladder. The ruptures of the *Umbilicus* and groin may be reſtrained and kept up by proper compreſſion, but it is very difficult to contrive an effectual bandage for the deſcent in the *Perineum*.

SECT.

SECT. III.

Of DROPSIES.

DIfficulty in breathing in pregnant women, may be occaſioned by collections of matter in the cheſt or *Thorax*, as well as in the *Abdomen*, from abſceſſes in the *Viſcera*, co-operating with the preſſure of the *Uterus* upon the organs of reſpiration: theſe complaints (which are generally fatal) muſt be treated by the ſame method in pregnancy which is uſed at other times. The cavity of the *Abdomen* is alſo ſubject to an *Aſcites* or dropſy, with or without *Hydatids*, which, in conjunction with the ſtretching *Uterus*, may diſtend the belly to a prodigious ſize, producing great oppreſſion and anxiety. Here too the common method of curing or palliating dropſies muſt be uſed, with this difference, that the purging medicines are to be cautiouſly preſcribed.

But this diſorder is not ſo incident to pregnant women as the *Anaſarca*, which is a dropſy of the cellular membrane, that extends over the whole ſurface of the body, invelloping every individual muſcle, veſſel, and fibre. This diſeaſe is the effect of univerſal laxity and weakneſs, and if not timely obviated, may endanger the patient's life, being ſometimes attended with a fatal rupture of the *Uterus* in time of labour: in order to prevent which cataſtrophe, every thing ought to be preſcribed in point of diet, medicine, and exerciſe, which may contribute to ſtrengthen the ſolids and quicken the circulation. Let her, for example, take repeated doſes of the *Confect. Cardiac.* drink moderate quantities of ſtrong wine, in which the warm ſpices have been infuſed, eat no meat but ſuch as is roaſted and high ſeaſoned, and abſtain altogether from weak diluting fluids, ſuch as ſmall beer and water.

SECT. IV.

Of incontinence of URINE, *and difficulty in making water at the latter end of pregnancy, and in time of labour.*

THE *Veſica urinaria* in pregnant women near their full time, is often ſo much preſſed by the *Uterus*, that it will contain but

but a very ſmall quantity of water; a circumſtance, though not dangerous, extremely troubleſome, eſpecially when attended with a vomiting or cough: in which caſe the ſtraining forces out the water involuntarily, with great violence. The cough may be alleviated by proper remedies, but the vomiting can ſeldom be removed; ſometimes a bandage applied round the lower part of the belly, and ſupported with the *Scapùlar*, is of ſingular ſervice, particularly when the *Uterus* lies pendulous over the *Os pubis*, thereby compreſſing the urinary bladder.

But this complaint is not of ſuch dangerous conſequence as a difficulty in making water, or a total ſuppreſſion, which (as we have already obſerved) happens, though very ſeldom, in the fourth or beginning of the fifth month of pregnancy; but moſt frequently occurs in time of labour, and after delivery. In the beginning of labour, before the membranes are broke, and the head of the child ſunk into the paſſage, the woman commonly labours under an incontinence of urine from the preſſure upon the bladder; but the membranes being broken,

and

and the waters diſcharged, the *Uterus* contracts, and the child's head is forced down into the *Pelvis,* where if it continues for any length of time, the *Urethra* or *Sphincter veſicæ* are ſo compreſſed that the urine cannot paſs; while the preſſure on the other parts of the bladder, being removed in conſequence of the diminiſhed ſize of the *Uterus*, and the laxity of the *Parietes* of the *Abdomen*, the *Veſica urinaria* is the more eaſily ſtretched by the increaſing quantity of urine; which diſtends it to ſuch a degree, that the fibres are over-ſtrained: and after delivery, when the preſſure is removed from the *Sphincter* and *Meatus urinarius*, it cannot contract ſo as to diſcharge its contents, eſpecially if any ſwelling or inflammation remains from the preſſure upon the neck and *Urethra*; in which caſe the patient is afflicted with violent ſtretching pains in the loins, back, groins, and particularly above the *Os pubis*.

This complaint is immediately removed by drawing off the urine with a catheter; and indeed this expedient ought to be tried before delivery, as it muſt infallibly promote labour,

labour, becauſe one pain interferes with the other. If the inflammation continues or increaſes, and the obſtruction of urine recurs after delivery, the external parts ought to be fomented with warm ſtupes, bladders half filled with warm water, or emollient decoctions may be applied as hot as the patient can bear them, to all the lower part of the belly, and the catheter be uſed twice a day, or as often as neceſſity requires, until the bladder ſhall have recovered its tone, ſo as to perform its office without aſſiſtance.

SECT. V.

Of the FLUOR ALBUS *in pregnant Women.*

THIS diſcharge, to which women are more ſubject at other times than during uterine geſtation, if in a large quantity, may hinder conception. In thoſe who are uſually troubled with it, the complaint generally ceaſes all the time of pregnancy: in ſome, however, it continues to the laſt, provided the ſeat of it is in the *Vagina*; and the evacuation is ſometimes ſo great, as to weaken both mother and child, and even to produce a miſcarriage. Every thing that ſtrengthens and nouriſhes the body is here of ſervice. This is alſo ſuppoſed to happen when ſome part of the *Chorion* being ſeparated from the *Uterus*, the fluid that is ſecreted by the *Colatura lactea* for the nutrition of the *Fœtus*, forces its way through the *Os internum*; and the greater this ſeparation is, and the nearer the full time, the larger the diſcharge will be.

SECT. VI.

Of the GONORRHEA *and* LUES VENEREA.

THOUGH women are not ſo ſoon infected with this diſtemper as men, they are commonly cured with greater difficulty, becauſe of the great moiſture and laxity of the parts affected; eſpecially in pregnant women, who nevertheleſs are to be treated in the ſame method practiſed at other times, except that in this caſe, mercurials and cathartics ought to be very cautouſly uſed: for if the *Gonorrhea* is neglected, or unſkilfully managed, the *Virus* will increaſe, and actually degenerate into a confirmed pox. It is often difficult to diſtinguiſh a *Gonorrhea* from the *Fluor Albus*, becauſe the colour and quantity of the diſcharge is nearly the ſame in both: in the laſt, however, we ſeldom meet with inflammation or ulcers within the *Labia* or entrance of the *Vagina*, whereas in the firſt theſe generally appear ſoon after the infection, about the *Meatus urinarius*, the *Carunculæ myrtiformes*, and inſide of the *Labia*, producing a violent pain in making water. The *Gonorrhea* is likewiſe diſtinguiſhed from the *Fluor Albus*, by its continuing all the time of the menſtrual diſcharge, during which the other complaint is commonly ſuſpended; but this mark is at beſt but uncertain, and can be of no ſervice in pregnancy, becauſe then the *Menſes* themſelves are obſtructed. The cure is beſt attained by bleeding, repeated doſes of gentle cathartics mixed with mercurials, a low diet, emulſions impregnated with nitre, and laſtly, balſamic, ſtrengthening, and aſtringent medicines.

If the diſtemper hath proceeded to an inveterate degree of the ſecond infection, attended with cancerous ulcerations of the *Pudenda*, bubos in the groin, ulcers in the noſe and throat, ſo that the life of the patient or conſtitution of the parts are endangered, mercurials muſt be given, ſo as to raiſe a gentle degree of ſalivation; which ought to be immediately reſtrained, and even carried off, by mild purgatives, and renewed occaſionally, according to the ſtrength of the woman, until the *Virus* be utterly diſcharged. Here, however, a great deal muſt depend upon the judgment and diſcretion of the preſcriber, who rather than propoſe any thing that might occaſion abortion, ought to try by palliating medicines to alleviate and keep under the ſymptoms till after delivery.

CHAP. III.

SECT. I.

Of MISCARRIAGES.

MOST of the complaints above deſcribed, if violent and neglected, may occaſion a miſcarriage; and it would be be almoſt an endleſs taſk to enumerate every accident from which this misfortune may proceed: I ſhall therefore content myſelf with deſcribing in what manner abortion happens; firſt, in the death of the child; ſecondly, in the ſeparation of the *Placenta*; and laſtly, in whatever may occaſion too great extenſion of the neck, and of the *Os internum*.

SECT. II.

Of the CHILD'S *Death.*

THIS may proceed from diſeaſes peculiar to itſelf, not to be accounted for, as well as from divers accidents that befal it in the womb: if, for example, the navel-ſtring be long, and the quantity of ſurrounding waters great, the *Fœtus* while young, may, in ſwimming, form a nooſe of the *Funis*, through which, if the head only paſſes, a circumvolution will happen round the neck or body: but ſhould the whole *Fœtus* paſs or thread this nooſe, a knot will be formed on the navel-ſtring, which if tight drawn, will abſolutely obſtruct the circulation. This may likewiſe be the caſe, when the waters are in very ſmall quantity, and the *Funis Umbilicalis* falls down before the head, by which it is violently compreſſed. In ſhort, the death of the *Fœtus* will be effected by all circumvolutions, knots, or preſſure upon the navel-ſtring, which deſtroy the circulation betwixt the *Placenta* and the child.

The *Fœtus* may ſuffer death from diſeaſes and accidents that happen to the mother; from violent paſſions of joy, fear or anger, ſuddenly raiſed to ſuch tranſports as occaſion tremors, fainting, or convulſions; and from a *Plethora*, and all acute diſtempers in which the circulating force of the fluids is too violent.

The child being dead, and the circulation in the ſecundines conſequently deſtroyed, the *Uterus* is no longer ſtretched, the *Fœtus* (if large) is no longer felt to move or ſtir; all the contained parts run gradually into a ſtate of putrefaction; the reſiſtance of the membranes becomes weaker than the contracting force of the *Uterus*, joined with the preſſure of the contents and parietes of the

Abdomen;

Abdomen; the contained waters of conſequence, burſt through their mortified incloſure, and the *Uterus* is contracted cloſe to its contents, which are therefore preſſed down lower and lower; the neck and mouth of the womb being gradually ſtretched, labour comes on, and a miſcarriage enſues.

At other times, gripings, looſeneſs and labour pains, even before the membranes break, are occaſioned by obſtruction or reſiſtance of the veſſels of the *Uterus*; in theſe caſes, if no flooding happens, the woman is ſeldom in danger, and though the child is known to be dead, the progreſs of nature is to be waited for with patience: if the woman is weak, exhauſted or timorous, ſhe muſt be encouraged and fortified with nouriſhing diet; if plethoric, ſhe muſt undergo evacuation by bleeding and laxative medicines, and when labour begins, be aſſiſted according to the directions ſpecified in the ſequel.

SECT. III.

Of the ſeparation of the PLACENTA *from the* UTERUS.

THIS ſeparation may proceed from all the foregoing diſeaſes and accidents that happen to the mother: from violent ſhocks, ſtrains, over-reachings, falls and bruiſes on the *Abdomen*; as alſo from vehement coughs, vomitings or ſtrainings at ſtool when the body is coſtive. The ſeparation of the *Placenta* is always accompanied with a diſcharge of blood from the veſſels of the *Uterus*, more or leſs, according to the term of pregnancy, or as the *Placenta* is more or leſs detached.

This diſcharge is diſtinguiſhed from the *Menſes* by the irregularity of its period, by its flowing in a larger quantity, and, after a ſmall intermiſſion, its return upon the leaſt motion of the patient.

The younger the woman is with child, the danger is the leſs; becauſe, though a conſiderable quantity of blood be loſt, it does not flow with ſuch violence as to exhauſt her immediately; and therefore, ſhe may be

ſupported

ſupported and her ſpirits kept up with proper cordials and nutritive diet. But when ſuch an hæmorrhage happens in any of the three or four laſt months of pregnancy, the danger is much more imminent, eſpecially towards the full time; becauſe the veſſels of the *Uterus* being then largely diſtended, a much greater quantity of blood is loſt in a ſhorter time; yet in both caſes, the flooding will be more or leſs, as there is more or leſs of the *Placenta* ſeparated from the womb; and when this happens in a very ſmall degree, the diſcharge may, by right management, be ſometimes ſtopped, and every thing will happily proceed to the full time; but if this purpoſe cannot be effected in a woman young with child, the principal intention ought to be a mitigation of the hæmorrhage, leaving the reſt to time and patience, as a miſcarriage in the firſt five months is ſeldom attended with hazard: on the contrary, nothing can be more dangerous than ſuch an effuſion in any of the four laſt months, provided it cannot be immediately reſtrained. In this caſe, we are often deceived by a ſhort intermiſſion, occaſioned by coagulated blood that locks up the

the mouth of the womb, which being pushed off, the flooding returns: and hence we account for its returning so commonly, upon motion, a fit of coughing, straining at stool, or any effort whatever.

It is happy for the woman, in this case, when she is so near the full time, that she may be sustained 'till labour is brought on; and this may be promoted, if the head presents, by gently stretching the mouth of the womb, which being sufficiently opened, the membranes must be broke; so that the waters being evacuated, the *Uterus* contracts, the flooding is restrained, and the patient safely delivered. At any rate, if the hæmorrhage returns again with great violence, there is no other remedy than that of delivering with all expedition, according to the method described in book III. chap. 4. sect. 3. and book IV. chap. 1. sect. 3.

Although the great danger is from floodings when near the full time; yet if labour can be brought on, the *Os Uteri* is easier dilated with the labour, or the hand; but in the sixth or seventh month, it takes longer time, and is stretched with greater difficul-

ty,

ty, which is ſometimes the occaſion of the danger at that period.

The edge or middle of the *Placenta* ſometimes adheres over the inſide of the *Os Internum*, which frequently begins to open ſeveral weeks before the full time; and if this be the caſe, a flooding begins at the ſame time, and ſeldom ceaſes intirely, until the woman is delivered: the diſcharge may indeed be intermitted by coagulums that ſtop up the paſſage, but when theſe are removed it returns with its former violence, and demands the ſame treatment that is recommended above.

In all caſes, and at all times of pregnancy, if the woman receives any extraordinary ſhock either in mind or body; if ſhe is attacked by a violent fever, or any complaints attending a *Plethora*, bleeding ought always to be preſcribed by way of prevention or precaution, unleſs a low, weak, lax habit of body renders ſuch evacuation unadviſeable; but theſe are not ſo ſubject to fevers from fullneſs.

On the firſt appearance of flooding, the patient ought immediately to be blooded to the amount of eight or twelve ounces, and venæſection repeated occaſionally, according to the ſtrength of the conſtitution, and emergency of the caſe: ſhe ought to be confined to her bed, and be rather cool than warm; if coſtive, an emollient glyſter muſt be injected, in order to diſſolve the hardened *Fæces*, that they may be expelled eaſily without ſtraining: internally, emulſions with nitre, muſt be uſed, and mixtures of the tinct. roſar. rub. acidulated with ſp. of vitriol, as the cooling or reſtringent method ſhall ſeem to be indicated; but above all things, opiates muſt be adminiſtred, to procure reſt, and quiet the uneaſy apprehenſions of the mind: for diet, let her uſe panada, weak broth, and rice gruel; ſhe may drink water in which a red hot iron has been ſeveral times quenched, mixed with a ſmall proportion of red burnt wine; ſhe muſt abſtain from all the high-ſeaſoned foods, and even fleſh meat or ſtrong broths, that will inrich the blood too faſt, and quicken the circulation. But if, notwithſtanding this regimen, the flooding ſhall continue and increaſe, ſo that the patient becomes faint and low, with

loſs

loſs of blood; we muſt, without further delay, attempt to deliver her, as in book III. chap. 9. ſect. 3. though this is ſeldom practicable, except in the laſt months of pregnancy, and then will be the eaſier performed the nearer ſhe is to her full time, unleſs labour pains ſhall have aſſiſted or begun a dilation of the *Os Internum*.

SECT. IV.

MISCARRIAGES may alſo be produced from every force that will ſtretch the neck and mouth of the womb; ſuch as violent coughs, vomitings, coſtive ſtrainings at ſtool, catharticks that bring on a ſuperpurgation, and teneſmus, together with frequent convulſions. All theſe ſymptoms muſt be treated in the uſual method: the cough and vomiting may be abated or removed chiefly by venæſection and opiates, the conſtipation by glyſters and gentle laxative medicines, the ſuperpurgation by opiates, the teneſmus by theſe and oily injections; the convulſions by blooding and bliſters; and as the more violent convulſions happen generally when the woman is near her full time, if they are not ſoon

ſoon removed, but continue and increaſe, to the manifeſt hazard of the patient's life, ſhe ought to be delivered immediately, in the ſame manner as in the caſe of a flooding in the laſt months.

SECT. V.

ABORTION may be likewiſe occaſioned by uncommon longings for things that cannot be ſoon or eaſily got, or ſuch as the woman is aſhamed to aſk for, eſpecially in her firſt child, namely different kinds of food and drink. Theſe appetites, if not gratified, ſometimes produce a miſcarriage, and indeed are ſuppoſed to affect the child in ſuch a manner, that the body of it ſhall be impreſſed with marks reſembling the figure or colour of what the mother longed for. Theſe cravings, therefore, though they appear unreaſonable and improper, muſt be ſatisfied, and the mother ought to ſhun every thing that is diſagreeable to the ſenſes, becauſe miſcarriage may alſo proceed from ſurprize at ſight of ſtrange and horrible objects.

BOOK

BOOK III.

CHAP. I.

SECT. I.

Of the CHILD'S *situation in the* UTERUS.

THE *Embrio* or *Fœtus*, as it lies in the *Uterus*, is nearly of a circular or rather oval figure, which is calculated to take up as little ſpace as poſſible: the chin reſts upon the breaſt, the thighs are preſſed along the belly, the heels applied to the breech, the face being placed between the knees, while the arms croſs each other, round the legs. The head for the moſt part, is down to the lower part of the *Uterus*; and the child being contracted into an oval form, the greateſt length is from head to breech: but the diſtance from one ſide to the other, is much leſs, than that from the

fore

fore to the back part; becauſe the thighs and legs are doubled along the belly and ſtomach, and the head bended forwards on the breaſt. The *Uterus* being confined by the *Vertebræ* of the loins, the diſtance from the back to the forepart of it, muſt be leſs than from ſide to ſide; ſo that, in all probability, one ſide of the *Fœtus* is turned towards the back, and the other to the forepart of the womb: but as the back part of the *Uterus* forms a little longiſh cavity on each ſide of the *Vertebræ*, the foreparts of the *Fœtus* may therefore, for the moſt part, tilt more backwards than forwards.

It has been generally ſuppoſed, that the head is turned up to the *Fundus*, and the breech to the *Os uteri*, with the foreparts towards the mother's belly; and that it remains in this ſituation till labour begins, when the head comes downwards, and the face is turned to the back of the mother. Some alledge, that the head precipitates about the end of the eighth or beginning of the ninth month, by becoming ſpecifically heavier than the reſt of the body. Others affirm, that as the child increaſes in bulk, eſpe-

eſpecially during the two laſt months, the proportion of ſurrounding water muſt be diminiſhed, ſo as that it is confined in its motion, and in ſtruggling to alter its poſition, the head is moved to the *Os tincæ*, where it remains till delivery. The particulars of this and other theories, may be found in *Mauriceau*, *La Motte*, *Simpſon* and *Old*. But from the following obſervations, it ſeems more probable, that the head is, for the moſt part, turned down to the lower part of the *Uterus*, from conception to delivery.

In the firſt month, according to ſome writers, the *Embryo* exhibits the figure of a tadpole, with a large head and ſmall body or tail, which gradually increaſes in magnitude, till the arms and thighs begin to bud or ſtrut out, like ſmall nipples, from the ſhoulders and breech: two black ſpecks appear on each ſide of the head, with a little hole or opening between them, which in the ſecond month, are eaſily diſtinguiſhed to be the eyes and mouth. The legs and arms are gradually formed, while the body turns larger, but the fingers are not ſeparated or diſtinct till the latter end of the ſecond, or beginning of the third month. This is commonly the caſe, but ſometimes, the bulk and appearance differ conſiderably in different *Embrios* of the ſame age. The younger the *Embrio*, the larger and heavier is the head in proportion to the reſt of the body, and this is the caſe in all the different gradations of the *Fœtus*; ſo that when dropt or ſuſpended by the navel-ſtring in water, the head muſt ſink lowermoſt, of courſe. Beſides, when women miſcarry, in the fourth, fifth, ſixth and ſeventh months, the head, for the moſt part, preſents itſelf, and is firſt delivered. By the touch in the *Vagina*, the head is frequently felt in the ſeventh, ſometimes in the ſixth, but more frequently in the eighth month; and if the ſame women are thus examined, trom time to time, till the labour begins, the head will always be felt of a round firm ſubſtance, at the fore part of the brim of the *Pelvis*, betwixt the *Os Internum* and *Pubis*, through the ſubſtance of the *Vagina* and *Uterus*. But all theſe opinions are liable to objections. If the deſcent of the head proceeded from its ſpecific gravity, we ſhould always find it at the *Os Internum*, becauſe this reaſon would always prevail: if it were owing to a diminiſhed proportion of water, why ſhould we often find the breech preſented, even when there is a quantity of that fluid large enough to give the head free liberty to riſe again towards the *Fundus*, or (according to the other opinion) to ſink down by its ſpecific gravity, to the *Os Internum?* Some, indeed, ſuppoſe, that the head always preſents itſelf, except when it is hindered by the *Funis Umbilicalis* twiſting round the neck and body, ſo as to impede the natural progreſs: but were this ſuppoſition juſt, when we turn and deliver by the feet thoſe children that preſented in a præternatural way, we ſhould always find them more or leſs circumvoluted by the navel-ſtring: whereas I have as often found the *Funis* twiſted round the neck and body, when the head preſented, as in any other caſe; and when other parts offered, have frequently delivered the child without finding it in the leaſt entangled by that cord. That the head is downwards all the time of geſtation, ſeems on the whole, to be the moſt reaſonable opinion, though it be liable to the objection already mentioned, and ſeems contradictory to the obſervation of ſome authors, who alledge, that in opening women that died in the fifth, ſixth, or ſeventh month, they have found the child's head towards the *Fundus Uteri*. But as it lies as eaſy in one poſture as in another, 'till the birth, this diſpute is of leſs conſequence in the practice of Midwifery.

SECT. II.

Of TOUCHING.

TOUCHING is performed by introducing the fore finger lubricated with pomatum, into the *Vagina*, in order to feel the *Os Internum* and neck of the *Uterus*; and ſometimes into the *Rectum*, to diſcover the ſtretching of the *Fundus*. By ſome we are adviſed to touch with the middle finger, as being the longeſt; and by others, to employ both that and the firſt; but the middle is too much encumbered by that on each ſide, to anſwer the purpoſe fully, and when two are introduced together, the patient never fails to complain. The deſign of touching is to be informed whether the woman

is,

is, or is not with child; to know how far ſhe is advanced in her pregnancy; if ſhe is in danger of a miſcarriage; if the *Os Uteri* be dilated; and in time of labour to form a right judgment of the caſe, from the opening of the *Os Internum*, and the preſſing down of the membranes with their waters; and laſtly, to diſtinguiſh what part of the child is preſented.

It is generally impracticable to diſcover by a touch in the *Vagina*, whether or not the *Uterus* is impregnated, 'till after the fourth month: then the beſt time for examination is the morning when the woman is faſting, after the contents of the bladder and *Rectum* have been diſcharged; and ſhe ought, if neceſſary, to ſubmit to the inquiry in a ſtanding poſture; becauſe in that caſe, the *Uterus* hangs lower down in the *Vagina*, and the weight is more ſenſible to the touch than when ſhe lies reclined. One principal reaſon of our uncertainty is, when we try to feel the neck, the womb riſes up on our preſſing againſt the *Vagina*, at the ſide of the *Os Internum*; and in ſome the *Vagina* feels very tenſe, but when the *Fundus Uteri* is advanced near the navel, the preſſure from above keeps down the *Os internum* ſo much, that you can generally feel both the neck, and, above that, the ſtretching of the under part of the *Uterus.*

There is no conſiderable variation to be felt in the figure of the *Os internum*, except in the latter end of pregnancy, when it ſometimes grows larger and ſofter; nor do the lips ſeem to be more cloſed in a woman with child than in another, eſpecially in the beginning of pregnancy: but in both caſes the *Os uteri* is felt like the mouth of a young puppy or tench, as we have before obſerved. In ſome the lips are very ſmall, in others large, and ſometimes, though ſeldom, ſmoothed over or pointed. In many women, who have formerly had children and difficult labours, the lips are large, and ſo much ſeparated, as to admit the tip of an ordinary finger; but a little higher up, the neck ſeems to be quite cloſed.

In the firſt four months, the neck of the womb may be felt hanging down in the *Vagina*, by puſhing up the finger by the ſide of the *Os internum*; but the ſtretching of the *Uterus* and upper part of the neck cannot be

per-

perceived till the fifth, and ſometimes the ſixth month; and even then the *Uterus* muſt be kept down by a ſtrong preſſure upon the belly.

The ſtretching of the *Fundus* is ſometimes felt by the finger introduced into the *Rectum*, before it can be perceived in the *Vagina*; becauſe in this laſt method, the *Uterus* recedes from the touch, and riſes too high to be accurately diſtinguiſhed, whereas the finger being introduced into the *Rectum*, paſſes along the back of the womb almoſt to the upper part of the *Fundus*, which in an unimpregnated ſtate, is felt flat on the back-part, and jetting out at the ſides; but the impregnated *Uterus* is perceived like a large round tumor.

About the fifth or ſixth month the upper part of the *Uterus* is ſo much ſtretched, as to riſe three or four inches above the *Os pubis*, or to the middle ſpace between that and the navel; ſo that, by preſſing the hand on the belly, eſpecially of lean women, it is frequently perceived; and if, at the ſame time, the index of the other hand be introduced in the *Vagina*, the neck will ſeem ſhortened, particularly at the fore-part and ſides, and, as I have already obſerved, the weight will be ſenſibly felt: but if the parietes of the *Abdomen* are ſtretched after eating, one may be deceived by the preſſure of the ſtomach, becauſe weight and preſſure are the ſame. But all theſe ſigns are more perceptible towards the latter end of pregnancy; and in ſome women the *Os internum* is felt a little open ſome weeks before the full time, though generally it is not opened till a few days before labour begins.

From the fifth to the ninth month, the neck of the *Uterus* becomes ſhorter and ſhorter, and the ſtretching of the womb grows more and more perceptible. In the ſeventh month the *Fundus* riſes as high as the navel, in the eight month, to the middle ſpace, betwixt the navel and *Scrobiculum cordis*; and in the ninth, even to the *Scrobiculum*, except in pendulous bellies: but all theſe marks may vary in different women; for when the belly is pendulous, the parts below the navel are much more ſtretched than thoſe above, and hang over the *Os pubis*; the *Fundus* will then be only equal to, or a little higher than the navel, at other times the *Uterus* will riſe in the latter end of the ſeventh or eighth month to the *Scrobiculum cordis*. The neck of the womb will in ſome be felt as long in the eighth as in others in the ſixth or ſeventh month. This variation ſometimes makes the examination of the *Abdomen* more certain than the touch of the *Vagina*; and ſo *vice verſa*. At other times we muſt judge by both.

SECT. III.

Of the ſigns of CONCEPTION, *and the equivocal ſigns of pregnant and obſtructed women.*

THE ſigns of pregnancy are to be diſtinguiſhed from thoſe that belong to obſtructions, by the touch in the *Vagina* and motion of the child in the fifth or ſixth month; ſometimes by the touch in the *Rectum*, before and after the fifth month, when the tumor of the *Abdomen* is plainly perceived.

Moſt women, a day or two before the irruption of the *Catamenia*, labour under complaints

plaints proceeding from a *Plethora*; ſuch as ſtretching pains in the back and loins, inſide of the thighs, breaſt, and head; a ſickneſs and oppreſſion at the ſtomach, and a fullneſs of all the *Viſcera* of the *Abdomen*: and all theſe ſymptoms abate, and gradually vaniſh, when the diſcharge begins and continues to flow. But if the woman be obſtructed by any accident or error in the non-naturals, all thoſe complaints continue and increaſe, and are hardly diſtinguiſhable from the ſymptoms of pregnancy, till the end of the fourth month; at which period, women with child grow better, and all the complaints of fullneſs gradually wear off; whereas thoſe who are only obſtructed, grow worſe and worſe, from the increaſe of the *Lentor* in the fluids, which will in time produce various and dangerous diſeaſes. The *Fundus uteri* in the obſtructed patient is not ſtretched, the diſorder in her ſtomach is not ſo violent as in a pregnant woman, and ſeldom accompanied with reachings; while the woman with child is afflicted with a reaching every morning, and ſubject to longings beſides. The firſt labours under a fullneſs

of

of the veſſels; the laſt, over and above this complaint, ſuffers an additional one from the diſtenſion of the *Uterus* by the impregnated *Ovum*. Obſtructions and pregnancy are both accompanied by a ſtretching fullneſs in the breaſts; but in the laſt only may be perceived the *Areola*, or brown ring, round the nipples, from which, in the laſt months, a thin ſerum diſtils: but this circle is not always ſo diſcernible as in the firſt pregnancy, and even then is uncertain, as well as the others.

About the fifth or ſixth month, the circumſcribed tumour or ſtretching of the *Uterus*, is felt above the *Os pubis*; and by this circumſcription and conſiſtence, eaſily diſtinguiſhed from the *Aſcites* or dropſy of the *Abdomen*: it is alſo rounder and firmer than thoſe ſwellings that accompany obſtructions, which proceed from a general fullneſs of the veſſels belonging to the ligaments and neighbouring *Viſcera*.

On the whole, the difficulty of diſtinguiſhing between obſtruction and pregnancy in the firſt months, is ſo great, that we ought to be cautious in giving our opinion; and never

pre-

preſcribe ſuch remedies as may endanger the fruit of the womb, but rather endeavour to palliate the complaints, until time ſhall diſcover the nature of the caſe; and always judge on the charitable ſide, when life or reputation is at ſtake.

In the fifth or ſixth month of uterine geſtation, by the touch in the *Vagina* we perceive the neck of the womb conſiderably ſhortened, and the ſtretching of the lower part of the *Uterus* is then ſenſibly felt between the mouth of the womb and the *Pubis*, and on each ſide of the neck.

In the ſeventh month, the head of the child is frequently felt reſting againſt the lower part of the *Uterus*, between the *Pubis* and *Os internum*; and being puſhed upwards towards the *Fundus*, ſinks down again by its own gravity. All theſe diagnoſticks are more plain and certain, the nearer the patient approaches to the time of delivery.

Sometimes the head is not felt till the eighth or ninth month, and in ſome few caſes, not till after the membranes are broke, when it is forced down by the contraction of the *Uterus*, and ſtrong labour-pains. This

cir-

circumstance may be owing to the head's resting above the basin, especially in a narrow *Pelvis*; or to the distention of its belly with air after death, by which the *Fœtus* being rendered specifically lighter than the surrounding waters, the body floats up to the *Fundus*, if there is a large quantity of fluid in the membranes: nor is the body always felt, when the child lies across the *Uterus*.

SECT. IV.

How to distinguish the false labour from the true, and the means to be used on that occasion.

IF the *Os uteri* remains close shut, it may be taken for granted, that the woman is not yet in labour, notwithstanding the pains she may suffer; with regard to which, an accurate inquiry is to be made, and if her complaints proceed from an overstretching fullness of the *Uterus*, or vessels belonging to the neighbouring parts, blooding in the arm or ancle, to the quantity of six or eight ounces, ought to be prescribed and repeated occasionally. If the pains are occasioned by a looſeneſs or *Diarrhœa*, it muſt be immediately reſtrained with *Opiates*, as in lib. II. chap. 3. ſect. 4. Cholic pains are diſtinguiſhed from thoſe of labour, by being chiefly confined to the belly, without going off and returning by diſtinct intervals: they are for the moſt part produced by *Fœces* too long retained in the *Colon*, or by ſuch *Ingeſta* as occaſion a rarefaction or expanſion of air in the inteſtines; by which they are violently ſtretched and vellicated. This complaint muſt be removed by opening glyſters, to empty the guts of their noxious contents; and this evacuation being performed, opiates may be adminiſtred to aſſwage the pains; either to be injected by the *Anus*, taken by the mouth, or applied externally, in form of *Epithem* or embrocation.

Sometimes the *Os internum* may be a little dilated, and yet it may be difficult to judge whether or not the patient be in labour; the caſe, however, may be aſcertained after ſome attendance, by theſe conſiderations: if the woman is not arrived at her full time; if no ſoft or glary *Mucus* hath been diſcharged from the *Vagina*; if the pains are limited to the region of of the belly, without extending to the back and inside of the thighs; if they are slight, and continue without intermission or increase; nay, if they have long intervals, and recur without force sufficient to push down the waters and membranes, or child's head, to open the *Os internum*; if this part be felt thick and rigid, instead of being soft, thin, and yielding, we may safely pronounce, that labour is not yet begun: and those alarms are to be removed as we have directed in the case of false or cholic pains. Besides, if the pulse be quick and strong, and the patient attacked by stitches in the sides, back, or head, blooding will be likewise necessary.

SECT. V.

The Division of LABOURS.

HIPPOCRATES, and almost all the writers upon this subject from his time to the fifteenth century, divided labour into two kinds; namely, natural and præternatural: the first comprehended those cases in which the head, others the head and breech presented, though the presentation of the head was always deemed the moſt natural; the other included all births in which any other part of the body firſt offered itſelf; and although they did not, like us, uſe a third diſtinction, they ſeem to have underſtood it in their practice: for among their chirurgical operations, we always find a chapter on the method of delivering dead children, by opening the head and extracting with the crotchet. At preſent labours are divided into natural, according to the ancients, when the head or breech preſents; laborious, when, notwithſtanding this ſituation of the child, the delivery goes on ſo tediouſly that the woman is in danger of loſing her life, unleſs ſhe is aſſiſted with the operator's hand, fillet, forceps, blunt hook, or crotchet; and præternatural, when neither head nor breech preſents; ſo that for the moſt part, there is a neceſſity for turning the child, and bringing it away by the feet. But the diviſion of labours hath been varied according to the opinions of different people: ſome think, that all thoſe caſes ought to be deemed præternatural, in which any part of the body (the head itſelf not excepted) preſents in an unuſual ufual way. Others affirm, that whatever part prefents, or however the pofture of the child may be, if it is delivered without any other affiftance than that of the labour-pains, the birth ought to be called natural; laborious, when in thefe cafes the child is born with difficulty; and præternatural, when lying acrofs the *Uterus*, it muft be turned and delivered by the feet.

For my own part, having in teaching found all thefe divifions liable to objections, I have followed a method which is more fimple than the others, and will fave abundance of repetition.

I call that a natural labour in which the head prefents, and the woman is delivered by her pains and the affiftance commonly given: but fhould the cafe be fo tedious and lingering, that we are obliged to ufe extraordinary force, in ftretching the parts, extracting with the forceps, or (to fave the mother's life) in opening the head and delivering with the crotchet, I diftinguifh it by the appellation of laborious: and in the præternatural, comprehend all thofe cafes in which the child is brought by the feet, or the body delivered before the head. Neither do I mind how the child preſents, ſo much as the way in which it is delivered: for there are caſes in which the head preſents, and for ſeveral hours we expect the child will be delivered in the natural way; but if the woman has not ſtrength enough to force down the child's head into the *Pelvis*, or in floodings, we are at length obliged to turn and bring it by the feet, becauſe it is ſo high that the forceps cannot be applied; and if the child is not large, nor the *Pelvis* narrow, it were pity to deſtroy the hopes of the parents, by opening the ſkull and extracting with the crotchet. In this caſe, therefore, although the child preſents in a natural way, we are obliged to turn and deliver it in the ſame manner as if the ſhoulder, breaſt, or back had preſented; and generally this operation is more difficult than in either of thoſe caſes, becauſe if the waters are all diſcharged, and the *Uterus* cloſe contracted round the *Fœtus*, it is more difficult to raiſe the head to the *Fundus*. When the breech preſents, we are frequently obliged to puſh it up and ſearch for the

the legs, which being found, we proceed to deliver the body, and laſtly the head.

For a farther illuſtration, and to inform young practitioners that difficult caſes do not frequently occur, ſuppoſe, of three thouſand women in one town or village, one thouſand ſhall be delivered in the ſpace of one year, and in nine hundred and ninety of theſe births, the child ſhall be born without any other than common aſſiſtance: fifty children of this number ſhall offer with the forehead turned to one ſide, at the lower part of the *Pelvis*, where it will ſtop for ſome time; ten ſhall come with the forehead turned towards the groin, or middle of the *Pubis*; five ſhall preſent with the breech, two or three with the face, and one or two with the ear; yet all theſe ſhall be ſafely delivered, and the caſe be more or leſs lingering and laborious, according to the ſize of the *Pelvis* and child, or ſtrength of the woman: of the remaining ten that make up the thouſand, ſix ſhall preſent with the head differently turned, and two with the breech; and theſe cannot be ſaved without ſtretching the parts, uſing the forceps or crotchet, or pushing up the child, in order to bring it by the feet; this necessity proceeding either from the weakness of the woman, the rigidity of the parts, a narrow *Pelvis*, or a large child, *&c.* the other two shall lie across, and neither head nor breech, but some other part of the body present, so that the child must be turned and delivered by the feet. Next year let us suppose another thousand women delivered in the same place, not above three, six, or eight, shall want extraordinary assistance; nay, sometimes, though seldom, when the child is young, or unusually small, and the mother has strong pains and a large *Pelvis*, it shall be delivered even in the very worst position, without any other help than that of the labour-pains.

As the head, therefore, presents right in nine hundred and twenty of a thousand labours, all such are to be accounted natural; those of the other seventy, that require assistance, may be deemed laborious; and the other ten, to be denominated laborious or præternatural, as they are delivered by the head or feet.

In

In order, therefore, to render this treatiſe as diſtinct as poſſible, for the ſake of the reader's memory, as well as of the dependance and connection of the different labours, they are divided in the following manner: that is accounted natural, in which the head preſents and the woman is delivered without extraordinary help; thoſe births are called laborious or nonnatural, when the head comes along with difficulty, and muſt be aſſiſted either with the hand in opening the parts, or with the fillet or forceps, or even when there is a neceſſity for opening and extracting it with the crotchet; and thoſe in which the child is brought by the breech or feet, are denominated præternatural, becauſe the delivery is performed in a præternatural way.

CHAP. II.

Of NATURAL LABOURS.

SECT. I.

Of the different Positions of Women in Labour.

IN almoſt all countries, the woman is allowed either to ſit, walk about, or reſt upon a bed, until the *Os uteri* is pretty much dilated by the gravitation of the waters, or (when they are in ſmall quantity) by the head of the *Fœtus*, ſo that delivery is ſoon expected; then ſhe is put in ſuch poſition as is judged moſt ſafe, eaſy, and convenient for that purpoſe: but the patient may be put upon labour too maturely, and bad conſequences will attend ſuch miſtakes.

Among the *Ægyptians*, *Græcians*, and *Romans*, the woman was placed upon an high ſtool; in *Germany* and *Holland* they uſe the chair which is deſcribed by *Daventer* and *Hieſter*; and for hot climates the ſtool is perfectly well adapted, but in northern

thern countries and cold weather, ſuch a poſition muſt endanger the patient's health.

In the *Weſt Indies* and ſome parts of *Britain*, the woman is ſeated on a ſtool made in form of a ſemicircle: in other places ſhe is placed on a woman's lap; and ſome kneeling on a large cuſhion, are delivered backwards.

In *France* the poſition is chiefly that of half ſitting and half lying, on the ſide or end of a bed; or the woman being in naked bed, is raiſed up with pillows or a bed-chair.

The *London* method is very convenient in natural and eaſy labours: the patient lies in bed upon one ſide, the knees being contracted to the belly, and a pillow put between them to keep them aſunder. But the moſt commodious method is to prepare a bed and a couch in the ſame room, a piece of oiled cloth or dreſſed ſheep-ſkin is laid acroſs the middle of each, over the under ſheet, and above this are ſpread ſeveral folds of linen, pinned, or tied with knittings to each ſide of the bed and couch; theſe are deſigned to ſpunge up the moiſture in time of labour and after delivery, while the oiled cloths or ſheep-ſkins below, preſerve the feather-bed from being wetted or ſpoiled: for this purpoſe, ſome people lay beſides upon the bed, ſeveral under-ſheets over one another, ſo that by ſliding out the uppermoſt every day, they can keep the bed dry and comfortable.

The couch muſt be no more than three feet wide, and provided with caſters; and the woman without any other dreſs than that of a ſhort or half ſhift, a linen ſkirt or petticoat open before, and a bed-gown, ought to lie down upon it, and be covered with cloaths according to the ſeaſon of the year. She is commonly laid on the left ſide, but in this particular ſhe is to conſult her own eaſe; and a large ſheet being doubled four times or more, one end muſt be ſlipt in below her breech, while the other hangs over the ſide of the couch, to be ſpread upon the knee of the accoucheur or midwife, who ſits behind her on a low ſeat: as ſoon as ſhe is delivered, this ſheet muſt be removed, a ſoft, warm cloth applied to the *Os externum*, and the pillow taken from betwixt her knees: ſhe then

then muſt be ſhifted with a clean, warm, half ſhift, linen-ſkirt, and bed-gown, and her belly kept firm with the broad head-band of the ſkirt, the ends of which are to be pinned acroſs each other. Theſe meaſures being taken, the couch muſt be run cloſe to the bed-ſide, and the patient gently moved from one to another; but if there is no couch, the bed muſt be furniſhed with the ſame apparatus. Some again, are laid acroſs the foot of the bed, to the head of which the cloaths are previouſly turned up till after delivery, when the woman's poſture is adapted, and then they are rolled down again to cover and keep her warm: by this expedient, the place of a couch is ſupplied, and the upper part of the bed preſerved ſoft and clean; whereas thoſe who are laid above the cloaths, muſt be taken up and ſhifted while the bed is put to rights; in which caſe they are ſubject to fainting, and to ſuch as are very much enfeebled this fatigue is often fatal.

Women are moſt eaſily touched, leaſt fatigued, and kept warmeſt, when they lie on one ſide; but if the labour ſhould prove tedious,

dious, the *Parisian* method ſeems moſt eligible; becauſe when the patient half ſits, half lies, the brim of the *Pelvis* is horizontal, a perpendicular line falling from the middle ſpace between the *Scrobiculum cordis* and navel, would paſs exactly through the middle of the baſin, as in book I. chap. 1. In this poſition, therefore, the weight of the waters, and, after the membranes are broke, that of the child's head, will gravitate downwards, and aſſiſt in opening the parts; while the contracting force of the abdominal muſcles and *Uterus*, is more free, ſtrong, and equal in this than in any other attitude. Wherefore, in all natural caſes, when the labour is lingering or tedious, this or any other poſition, ſuch as ſtanding or kneeſing, ought to be tried; which by an additional force, may help to puſh along the head and alter its direction, when it does not advance in the right way. Nevertheleſs, the patient muſt by no means be too much fatigued.

When the woman lies on the left ſide, the right hand muſt be uſed in touching, and *vice verſa*, unleſs ſhe is laid acroſs the bed;

bed; in which caſe, either hand will equally anſwer the ſame purpoſe: but if ſhe lies athwart, with the breech towards the bed's foot, it will be moſt convenient to touch with the left hand when ſhe is upon the left ſide, and with the right when in the oppoſite poſition. And here it will not be amiſs to obſerve, that in the deſcription of all the laborious and præternatural deliveries treated of in this performance, the reader muſt ſuppoſe the woman lying on her back, as in chap. 3. ſect. 3. and chap. 4. ſect. 4. except when another poſture is preſcribed; and that in natural and laborious labours, whether ſhe be upon her ſide or back, the head and ſhoulders are a little raiſed into a reclining poſture, ſo that ſhe may breathe eaſily, and aſſiſt the pains.

But in præternatural labours, when there is a neceſſity for uſing great force in turning the child, the head and ſhoulders muſt lie lower than the breech; which being cloſe to the ſide or foot of the bed, ought to be raiſed higher than either, becauſe when the *Pelvis* is in this ſituation, the hand and arm are eaſier puſhed up in a right line, along the

the back-part of the *Uterus*, even to its *Fundus*. Sometimes, however, when the feet of the child are towards the belly of the mother, they are more eaſily felt and managed when ſhe lies on her ſide. At other times, placing the woman on her knees and elbows on a low couch, according to *Daventer*'s method, will ſucceed better, by diminiſhing in part the ſtrong reſiſtance from the preſſure and weight of the *Uterus* and child; by which the feet will ſometimes be eaſier found and delivered: but then it is ſafer for the child, and eaſier to the operator and mother, to turn her to her back before you deliver the body and head.

SECT. II.

Of the management of women in a NATURAL LABOUR.

IN a woman come to full time, labour commonly begins and proceeds in the following manner.

The *Os uteri* is felt ſoft and a little opened, the circumference being ſometimes thick,

thick, but chiefly thin; from this aperture is diſcharged a thick *Mucus*, which lubricates the parts and prepares them for ſtretching. This diſcharge uſually begins ſome days before, and is accounted the forerunner of real labour: at the ſame time the woman is ſeized at intervals with ſlight pains that gradually ſtretch the *Os uteri*, fitting it for a larger dilatation; and when labour actually begins, the pains become more frequent, ſtrong, and laſting.

At every pain the *Uterus* is ſtrongly compreſſed by the ſame effort which expels the contents of the *Rectum* at ſtool, namely, the inflation of the lungs, and the contraction of the abdominal muſcles.

If the child be ſurrounded with a large quantity of waters, the *Uterus* cannot come in contact with the body of it, but at every pain the membranes are puſhed down by the fluid they contain, and the mouth of the womb being ſufficiently opened by this gradual and repeated diſtention, they are forced into the middle of the *Vagina*; then the *Uterus* contracts, and comes in contact with the body of the child, and if it be ſmall,

the

the head is propelled with the waters. Here the membranes uſually break, but if that is not the caſe, they are puſhed along towards the *Os externum*, which they alſo gradually open, and appear on the outſide in the form of a large round bag: mean while the head advances, and the *Os externum* being by this time fully dilated, is alſo protruded; when, if the membranes, inſtead of burſting in the middle of the protuberance, are tore all round at the *Os externum*, the child's head is covered with ſome part of them, which goes under the name of the caul, or king's hood. If the *Placenta* is, at the ſame time, ſeparated from the *Uterus*, and the membranes remain unbroken, the ſecundines, waters, and child, are delivered together; but if the *Placenta* adheres, they muſt of courſe give way: and ſhould they be tore all round from the *Placenta*, the greateſt part of the body, as well as the head of the child, will be invelloped by them, from which it muſt be immediately diſengaged, that the air may have a free paſſage into the lungs.

When the head is large, ſo that it does not deſcend immediately into the *Pelvis*, the mem-

membranes are forced down by themſelves; and being ſtretched thinner and thinner, give way; when all the waters which are farther advanced than the head run out; then the *Uterus* coming in contact with the body of the child, the head is ſqueezed down into the mouth of the womb, which it plugs up ſo as to detain the reſt of the waters.

Sometimes, when the quantity of waters is very ſmall, and the *Uterus* embraces the body of the child, the head, covered with the membranes, is forced downwards, and gradually opens the *Os internum*; but at its arrival in the middle of the *Pelvis* and *Vagina*, part of the waters will be puſhed down before it, ſometimes in a large, and ſometimes in a ſmall proportion, towards the back-part of the *Pelvis*. At other times, when the waters are in ſmall quantity, no part of them are to be diſtinguiſhed farther than the head, which deſcending lower and lower, the attenuated membranes are ſplit upon it; while, at the ſame time, it fills up the mouth of the womb and upper part of the *Vagina*, in ſuch a manner as hinders the

few

few remaining waters from being discharged at once; though in every pain a small quantity distils on each side of the head, for lubricating the parts, so as that the child may slip along the more easily.

The *Uterus* contracts, the pains become quicker and stronger, the crown of the head is pushed down to the lower part of the *Pelvis*, against one of the *Ischia*, at its lower extremity; the forehead being at the upper part of the opposite *Ischium*, is forced into the hollow of the under part of the *Sacrum*, while the *Vertix* and hindhead is pressed below the *Os pubis*; from whence it rises in a quarter turn, gradually opening the *Os externum*: the *Frænum labiorum*, or *Fourchette*, *Perinæum*, fundament, and the parts that intervene betwixt that and the extremity of the *Sacrum*, are all stretched outwards in form of a large tumor. The *Perinæum*, which is commonly but one inch from the *Os externum* to the *Anus*, is now stretched to three, the *Anus* to two, and the parts between that and the *Coccyx* are stretched from two inches to about three or more. The broad *Sacrosciatic* ligaments reaching from each

each ſide of the lower part of the *Sacrum*, to the under part of each *Iſchium*, are alſo outwardly extended, and the *Coccyx* is forced backward; while the crown of the head, where the lambdoidal croſſes the end of the ſagittal ſuture, continues to be puſhed along, and dilates the *Os externum* more and more.

When the head is ſo far advanced, that the back-part of the neck is come below the under-part of the *Pubis*, the forehead forces the *Coccyx*, fundament, and *Perinæum* backwards and downwards; then the hindhead riſes about two or three inches from under the *Pubis*, making an half-round turn in its aſcent, by which the forehead is equally raiſed from the parts upon which it preſſed, and the *Perinæum* eſcapes without being ſplit or torn: at the ſame time, the ſhoulders advance into the ſides of the *Pelvis* at its brim, where it is wideſt, and, with the body, are forced along and delivered; mean while, by the contraction of the *Uterus*, the *Placenta* and *Chorion* are looſened from the inner ſurface to which they adhered, and forced through the *Vagina*, out at the *Os externum*.

When the head reſts at firſt above the brim of the *Pelvis*, and is not far advanced, the *Fontanelle* may be plainly felt with the finger, commonly towards the ſide of the *Pelvis:* this is the place where the coronal croſſes the ſagittal ſuture, and the bones are a little ſeparated from each other, yielding a ſoftneſs to the touch, by which may be diſtinguiſhed four ſutures, or rather one croſſing another. Theſe may be plainly perceived, even before the membranes are broke, yet the examination muſt not be made during a pain, when the membranes are ſtretched down and filled with waters; but only when the pain begins to remit, and the membranes to be relaxed, otherwiſe they may be broke too ſoon, before the *Os internum* is ſufficiently dilated, and the head properly advanced.

When the *Vertix* is come lower down, the ſagittal ſuture only is to be felt; becauſe as the hindhead deſcends in the *Pelvis*, the *Fontanelle* is turned more backwards, to the ſide, or towards the concavity of the *Sacrum:* but after it has arrived below the under part of the *Pubis*, the lambdoidal

may

may be felt croſſing the end of the ſagittal ſuture, the *Occiput* making a more obtuſe angle than that of the parietal bones, at the place where the three are joined together. But all theſe circumſtances are more eaſily diſtinguiſhed after the membranes are broke, or when the head is ſo compreſſed that the bones ride over one another, provided the hairy ſcalp be not exceſſively ſwelled.

SECT. III.

How to behave when the birth is obſtructed by the navel-ſtring or ſhoulders of the child. Vide book II. *chap.* 2. *ſect.* 3.

ALthough the head is puſhed down into the *Pelvis*, and the *Vertix* employed in opening the *Os externum*, the forehead being lodged in the concavity formed by the *Coccyx* and lower part of the *Sacrum*; yet frequently after the labour-pain is abated, the head is again withdrawn by the navel-ſtring happening to be twiſted round the neck; or when the ſhoulders, inſtead of advancing, are retarded at the brim of the *Pelvis*, one reſting over the *Pubis*, while the

the other is fixed at the *Sacrum*; or when (the waters having been long evacuated) the under-part of the *Uterus* contracts round the neck and before the ſhoulders, keeping up the body of the child.

When the head is therefore drawn back by any of theſe obſtacles, and the delivery hath been retarded during ſeveral pains, one or two fingers being introduced into the *Rectum* before the pain goes off, ought to preſs upon the forehead of the child at the root of the noſe, great care being taken to avoid the eyes: this preſſure detains the head till the return of another pain, which will ſqueeze it farther down, while the fingers puſhing ſlowly and gradually, turn the forehead half round outwards and half round upwards. By this aſſiſtance, and the help of ſtrong pains, the child will be forced along, although the neck be entangled in the navel-ſtring; for as the child advances, the *Uterus* contracts, and conſequently the *Placenta* is moved lower: the *Funis umbilicalis* will alſo ſtretch a little, without obſtructing the circulation.

The

The head being thus kept down, the ſhoulders too are preſſed in every ſucceeding pain, until they are forced into the *Pelvis*, when the whole comes along, without further difficulty. And this expedient will, moreover, anſwer the purpoſe, when the under-part of the *Uterus* or *Os internum* is contracted round the neck of the child, and before the ſhoulders; alſo when the head is very low, preſſing a finger on each ſide of the *Coccyx* externally, will frequently aſſiſt in the ſame manner.

Over and above theſe obſtacles, the head may be actually delivered and the body retained by the contraction of the *Os externum* round the neck, even after the face appears externally. In this caſe it was generally alledged, that the neck was cloſe embraced by the *Os internum*; but this ſeldom happens when the head is delivered, becauſe then the *Os internum* is kept dilated on the back-part and ſides by the breaſt and arms of the *Fœtus*, unleſs it be forced low down with or before the head.

When the head is delivered, and the reſt of the body retained from the largeneſs or wrong preſenting of the ſhoulders, or by the navel-ſtring's being twiſted round the body or neck of the child, the head muſt be graſped on each ſide, the thumbs being applied to the *Occiput*, the fore and middle fingers extended along each ſide of the neck, while the third and fourth of each hand ſupport each ſide of the upper jaw; thus embraced, the head muſt be pulled ſtreight forwards, and if it will not move eaſily along, the force muſt be increaſed, and the direction varied from ſide to ſide, or rather from ſhoulder to ſhoulder, not by ſudden jirks, but with a ſlow, firm, and equal motion. If the body cannot be moved in this manner, though you have exerted as much force as poſſible, without running the riſk of over-ſtraining the neck, you muſt endeavour to ſlip the turns of the navel-ſtring over the head: but ſhould this be found impracticable, you ought not to trifle in tying the ſtring at two places, and cutting betwixt the ligatures, as ſome people have adviſed: ſuch an operation would engroſs too much time; beſides, the child is in no danger of ſuffocation from the

ſtricture

ſtricture of the *Funis*, becauſe it ſeldom or never breathes before the breaſt is delivered.

The better method is, immediately to ſlide along one or two fingers, either above or below, to one of the arm-pits; by which you try to bring along the body, while, with the other hand, you pull the neck at the ſame time: if it ſtill continues unmoved, ſhift hands, and let the other arm-pit ſuſtain the force; but if this fail, cut the navel-ſtring, and tie it afterwards. If the ſhoulders lie ſo high that the fingers cannot reach far enough to cut or take ſufficient hold, let the flat of the hand be run along the back of the child; or ſhould the *Os externum* be ſtrongly contracted round the neck, puſh up your hand along the breaſt, and pull as before: and ſhould this method fail, you muſt have recourſe to the blunt hook, introduced and fixed in the arm-pit; but this expedient muſt be uſed with caution, leſt the child ſhould be injured or the parts lacerated.

The child being born, the *Funis umbilicalis* muſt be divided, and the *Placenta* delivered, according to the directions that will occur in the ſequel.

SECT. IV.

How and when to break the MEMBRANES.

I Have already obſerved, that if the child be ſurrounded with a large quantity of waters, the *Uterus* cannot come in contact with the body ſo as to preſs down the head, until the membranes are puſhed a conſiderable way before it into the *Vagina*; nor even then, until they are broke, and the fluid diminiſhed in ſuch a manner as will allow the womb to contract, and, with the aſſiſtance of the pains, force along the child. When the membranes, therefore, are ſtrong or unadvanced, and continue ſo long unbroke, that the delivery is retarded, provided the *Os internum* be ſufficiently dilated, they ought to be broke without further delay; eſpecially if the woman hath been much fatigued or exhauſted with labour, or is ſeized with a violent flooding: in which caſe, the rupture of the membranes haſtens delivery, and the hæmorrhage is diminiſhed by the contraction of the *Uterus*, which leſ-

ſens

ſens the mouths of the veſſels that are alſo compreſſed by the body of the child.

The common method of breaking the membranes is by thruſting the finger againſt them when they are protruded with the waters during the pain, or by pinching them with the finger and thumb; but if they are detained too high to be managed in either of theſe methods, the hand may be introduced into the *Vagina*, if the *Os externum* is ſo lax as to admit it eaſily: and if this cannot be done without giving much pain, the fore and middle fingers being puſhed into the *Vagina* with the other hand, let a probe or pair of pointed ſciſſars be directed along and between them, and thruſt through the membranes, when they are puſhed with the waters, below the head. This operation muſt be cautiouſly performed, leſt the head ſhould be wounded in the attempt; and as for the membranes, let the opening be never ſo ſmall, the waters are diſcharged with force ſufficient to tear them aſunder.

SECT.

SECT. V.

NUMB. I.

When the Vertix *presents, and when little or no waters are protruded thereby.*

IF the *Vertix*, instead of resting at the side of the brim of the *Pelvis*, or at the *Os pubis*, is forced farther down to the *Os internum*, and the waters happen to be in small quantity, the head is pushed forwards, and gradually opens the mouth of the womb without any sensible interposition of the waters; then it advances by degrees into the *Vagina*, and the membranes being split or tore, little or nothing is discharged until the body of the child be delivered; and in this case, the hair of the head being plainly felt, will be a sufficient indication that the membranes are broke. If no hair is to be felt, but a smooth body presents itself to the touch, and the woman has undergone many strong pains, even after the mouth of the womb hath been largely dilated, and the head forced into the middle of the *Pelvis*, you

you may conclude, that delivery is retarded by the rigidity of the membranes, that there is but a ſmall quantity of waters, and that if the containing *Sacs* were broke, the head would come along, without further heſitation.

Sometimes no waters can be felt while the head is no farther advanced than the upper part of the *Pelvis*, becauſe it plugs up the paſſage and keeps them from deſcending; but as it advances downwards, the *Uterus* contracts, and they are forced down in a ſmall quantity towards the back-part: from thence, as the head deſcends, or even though it ſhould ſtick in that ſituation, they are puſhed farther down, and the membranes may be eaſily broke; but the taſk is more difficult when no waters come down, and the membranes are contiguous to the head. In this caſe, they muſt be ſcratched a little during every pain with the nail of a finger, which, though ſhort and ſmooth, will by degrees wear them thinner and thinner, until they ſplit upon the head by the force of labour. Yet this expedient ought never to be uſed until you are certain that delivery is retarded by their rigidity; for if that be not the hindrance, the difficulty muſt proceed from the weakneſs of the woman, a large head, or narrow *Pelvis:* in which caſe the delivery is a work of time, and will be obſtructed by the premature diſcharge of the waters, which, by gradually paſſing by the head, ought to keep the parts moiſt and ſlippery, in order to facilitate the birth; for when the membranes are not broke, until the head is forced into the middle of the *Pelvis*, the largeſt part of it being then paſt the upper part of the *Sacrum*, is commonly ſqueezed along, opens the *Os externum*, and is delivered before all the waters are diſcharged from the *Uterus*; ſo that what remains, by moiſtening and lubricating the parts, help the ſhoulders and body to paſs with more eaſe. When the membranes are too ſoon broke, the under-part of the *Uterus* contracts ſometimes ſo ſtrongly before the ſhoulders, that it makes the reſiſtance ſtill greater.

NUMB. II.

How to manage when the forehead is turned to one ſide.

IN moſt natural labours, the ſpace betwixt the fore and back *Fontanelles*, viz. the *Vertix*, preſents to the *Os internum*, and the forehead is turned to the ſide of the *Pelvis*; becauſe the baſin at the brim is wideſt from ſide to ſide, and frequently, before the head is puſhed in and faſt wedged among the bones, the child (after a pain) is felt to move and turn it to that ſide or ſituation in which it is leaſt preſſed and hurt, if it was not preſenting in that poſition before: but this poſition of the head may alter, viz. in thoſe where it is as wide, or wider, from the back-part to the fore-part of the brim, than from ſide to ſide, the forehead may be turned backwards or forewards. But this form of the *Pelvis* ſeldom happens.

This poſture is always obſerved in a narrow *Pelvis*, when the upper part of the *Sacrum* jets forward to the *Pubis*; but as the child is forced lower down, the forehead turns into the hollow at the inferior part of of the *Sacrum*, becauſe the *Vertix* and *Occiput* find leſs reſiſtance at the lower part of the *Pubis* than at the *Iſchium* to which it was before turned, the *Pelvis* being at the *Pubis*, as formerly deſcribed, no more than two inches in depth, whereas at the *Iſchium* it amounts to four. If, therefore, the forehead ſticks in its former ſituation, without turning into the hollow, it may be aſſiſted by introducing ſome fingers, or the whole hand, into the *Vagina*, during a pain, and moving it into the right poſition.

When the head of the *Fœtus* preſents, and is forced along in any of thoſe poſitions, the labour is accounted natural, and little elſe is to be done, but to encourage the woman to bear down with all her ſtrength in every pain, and to reſt quietly during each interval: if the parts are rigid, dry, or inflamed, they ought to be lubricated with *Pomatum*, hog's lard, butter, or *Ung. altheæ*; the two firſt are moſt proper for the external parts, and the two laſt (as being harder and not ſo eaſily melted) ought to be put up into the *Vagina*, to lubricate that and the *Os internum*.

NUMB.

NUMB. III.

How to aſſiſt in LINGERING LABOUR.

THE mouth of the womb and *Os externum*, for the moſt part, open with greater difficulty in the firſt than in the ſucceeding labours, more eſpecially in women turned of thirty. In theſe caſes, the *Os externum* muſt be gradually dilated in every pain, by introducing the fingers in form of a cone, and turning them round, ſo as to ſtretch the parts by gentle degrees; and the whole hand being admitted into the *Vagina*, it will be ſometimes found neceſſary to inſinuate the fingers with the flat of the hand between the head and *Os internum*: for when this precaution is not taken in time, the *Os uteri* is frequently puſhed before the head (eſpecially that part of it next the *Pubis*) even through the *Os externum*; or if the head paſſes the mouth of the womb, it will protrude the parts at the *Os externum*, and will endanger a laceration in the *Perinæum*. This dilatation, however, ought to be cautiouſly performed, and never attempted except when it is abſolutely neceſſary; even then it muſt

be

be effected ſlowly, and in time of a pain, when the woman is leaſt ſenſible of the dilating force.

When the labour happens to be lingering, though every thing be in a right poſture, if the aſſiſtants are clamorous, and the woman herſelf too anxious and impatient to wait the requiſite time, without complaining, the labour will be actually retarded by her uneaſineſs, which we muſt endeavour to ſurmount by arguments and gentle perſuaſion; but if ſhe is not to be ſatisfied, and ſtrongly impreſſed with an opinion, that certain medicines might be adminiſtred to haſten delivery, it will be convenient to preſcribe ſome innocent *Placemus*, that ſhe may take between whiles, to beguile the time and pleaſe her imagination: but if ſhe is actually weak and exhauſted, it will be neceſſary to order ſomething that will quicken the circulating fluids, ſuch as preparations of amber, caſtor, myrrh, volatile ſpirits, the pulv. myrrh. compoſit. of the *London*, or pulv. *ad partum* of the *Edinburgh Pharmacopeia*, with every thing in point of diet and drink that nouriſhes and ſtrengthens the body. If the patient is of a plethoric habit, with a quick, ſtrong pulſe, the contrary method is to be uſed, ſuch as venæſection, antiphlogiſtic medicines, and plentiful draughts of weak, diluting fluids.

SECT. VI.

NUMB. I.

How to manage the CHILD *after* DELIVERY.

THE Child being delivered, ought to be kept warm beneath the bed-cloaths, or immediately covered with a warmed flannel or linnen-cloth: if it cries and breathes, the umbilical cord may be tied and cut, and the child delivered to the nurſe without delay; but if the air does not immediately ruſh into the lungs, and the circulation continues between it and the *Placenta*, the operation of tying and cutting muſt be delayed, and every thing tried to ſtimulate and ſome times to give pain. If the circulation is languid, reſpiration begins with difficulty, and proceeds with long intervals; and if it be entirely ſtopped in the *Funis*, the child, if alive, is not eaſily recovered: ſometimes a great many minutes are elapſed before it begins to breathe. Whatever augments the circulating force, promotes reſpiration, and as this increaſes, the circulation grows ſtronger, ſo that they mutually aſſiſt each other. In order to promote the one and the other, the child is kept warm, moved, ſhaken, whipt; the head, temples, and breaſt, rubbed with ſpirits, garlick, onion, or muſtard applied to the mouth and noſe; and the child has been ſometimes recovered by blowing into the mouth with a ſilver *Canula*, ſo as to expand the lungs.

When the *Placenta* is itſelf delivered, immediately or ſoon after the child, by the continuance of the labour pains, or hath been extracted by the operator, that the *Uterus* may contract, ſo as to reſtrain too great a flooding; in this caſe, if the child has not yet breathed, and a pulſation is felt in the veſſels, ſome people (with good reaſon) order the *Placenta*, and as much as poſſible of the navel-ſtring, to be thrown into a baſin of warm wine or water, in order to promote the circulation between them and the child; others adviſe us to lay the *Placenta* on the

child's

child's belly, covered with a warm cloth; and a third ſet order it to be thrown upon hot aſhes: but of theſe, the warm water ſeems the moſt innocent and effectual expedient. Nevertheleſs, if the *Placenta* is ſtill retained in the *Uterus*, and no dangerous flooding enſues, it cannot be in a place of more equal warmth, while the operator endeavours, by the methods above deſcribed, to bring the child to life.

NUMB. II.

IN lingering labours, when the head of the child hath been long lodged in the *Pelvis*, ſo that the bones ride over one another, and the ſhape is præternaturally lengthened, the brain is frequently ſo much compreſſed, that violent convulſions enſue before or ſoon after the delivery, to the danger and oft-times the deſtruction of the child. This diſorder is frequently relieved and carried off, and the bad conſequences of the long compreſſion prevented, by cutting the navel-ſtring before the ligature is made, or tying it ſo ſlightly as to allow two, three, or four large ſpoonfuls to be diſcharged.

If the child has been dead one or two days before delivery, the lips and genitals (eſpecially the *Scrotum* in boys) are of a livid hue; if it hath lain dead in the *Uterus* two or three days longer, the ſkin may be eaſily ſtript from every part of the body, and the navel-ſtring appears of the ſame colour with the lips and genitals: in ten or fourteen days, the body is much more livid and mortified, and the hairy ſcalp may be ſeparated with eaſe; and indeed, any part of the child which hath been ſtrongly preſſed into the *Pelvis*, and retained in that ſituation for any length of time, will adopt the ſame mortified appearance.

NUMB. III.

How to tie the FUNIS UMBILICALIS.

DIFFERENT practitioners have uſed different methods of performing this operation: ſome propoſing to tie and ſeparate the *Funis* before the *Placenta* is delivered; to apply one ligature cloſe to the belly of the child, with a view to prevent a rupture of the navel; and making another two inches above the former, to divide the rope between the

two

two tyings: by the ſecond ligature, they mean to prevent a dangerous hæmorrhage from the woman, provided the *Placenta* adheres to the *Uterus*. But all theſe precautions are founded upon miſtaken notions, and the following ſeems to be that which is eaſieſt and beſt: if the *Placenta* is not immediately delivered by the pains, and no flooding obliges you to haſten the extraction, the woman may be allowed to reſt a little, and the child to recover; if it does not breathe, or the reſpiration is weak, let the methods above preſcribed be put in practice, with a view to ſtimulate the circulation; but if the child is lively, and cries with vigour, the *Funis* may be immediately tied in this manner; having provided a ligature or two, compoſed of ſundry threads waxed together, ſo as to equal the diameter of a packthread, being ſeven inches in length and knotted at each end, tie the navel ſtring about two fingers breadth from the belly of the child, by making at firſt one turn, if the *Funis* be ſmall, and ſecuring it with two knots; but if the cord be thick, make two more turns and another double knot, then cut the *Funis* with a pair of ſharp ſciſſars one finger's breadth from the ligature towards the *Placenta*; and in cutting, run the ſciſſars as near as poſſible to the root of the blades, elſe the *Funis* will be apt to ſlip from the edge, and you will be obliged to make ſeveral ſnips before you can effect a ſeparation: at the ſame time guard the points of the ſciſſars with your other hand. The child being waſhed, a linnen rag is wrapped round the tied *Funis*, which being doubled up along the belly, a ſquare compreſs is laid over it, and kept firm or moderately tight with what the nurſes call a belly-band, or roller round the body.

This portion of the *Funis* ſoon ſhrinks, turns firſt livid, then black, and about the fifth day falls off cloſe to the belly; and let the navel-ſtring be tied in any part, or at any diſtance whatſoever from the belly, it will always drop off at the ſame place: ſo that ruptures in the navel do not always depend upon the tying of the *Funis*, but may happen when the compreſs and belly-band are not kept ſufficiently firm, and continued ſome time after the ſeparation of the wither'd

portion,

portion, eſpecially in thoſe children that cry much: the bandage ought always to be applied ſo ſlight, as not to affect reſpiration.

The ligature upon the *Funis* muſt always be drawn ſo tight as to ſhut up the mouths of the veſſels; therefore if they continue to pour out their contents, another ligature muſt be applied below the former; for if this precaution be neglected, the child will ſoon bleed to death: yet, if the navel-ſtring is cut or tore aſunder at two or three hand-breadths from the belly, and expoſed to the cold without any ligature, the arteries will contract themſelves, ſo as that little or no blood ſhall be loſt; nay, ſometimes, if the *Funis* hath been tied and cut at the diſtance of three finger-breadths from the child's belly, ſo as that it hath been kept from blooding for an hour or two, although the ligature be then untied, and the navel-ſtring and belly chafed, and ſoaked in warm water, no more blood will be diſcharged.

SECT. VII.

Of delivering the PLACENTA.

THE *Funis* being ſeparated, and the child committed to the nurſe, the next care is to deliver the *Placenta* and membranes, if they are not already forced down by the labour-pains. We have already obſerved, that if there is no danger from a flooding, the woman may be allowed to reſt a little, in order to recover from the fatigue ſhe has undergone; and that the *Uterus* may, in contracting, have time to ſqueeze and ſeparate the *Placenta* from its inner ſurface: during which pauſe alſo, about one, two, or three tea-cups full of blood is diſcharged through the *Funis*, from the veſſels of the *Placenta*, which is thus diminiſhed in bulk, ſo that the womb may be the more contracted; and this is the reaſon for applying one ligature only upon the cord. In order to deliver the *Placenta*, take hold of the navel-ſtring with the left hand, turning it round the fore and middle fingers, or wrapping it in a cloth, that it may not ſlip from your

graſp;

graſp; then pull gently from ſide to ſide, and deſire the woman to aſſiſt your endeavour, by ſtraining as if ſhe were at ſtool, blowing forcibly into her hand, or provoking herſelf to reach by thruſting her finger into her throat. If by theſe methods the *Placenta* cannot be brought away, introduce your hand ſlowly into the *Vagina* and feel for the edge of the cake, which when you have found, pull it gradually along; as it comes out at the *Os externum*, take hold of it with both hands and deliver it, bringing away at the ſame time all the membranes, which, if they adhere, muſt be pulled along with leiſure and caution.

When the *Funis* takes it origin towards the edge of the *Placenta*, which is frequently the caſe, the cake comes eaſier off by pulling, than when the navel-ſtring is inſerted in the middle, unleſs it be uncommonly retained by its adheſion to the womb, or by the ſtrong contraction of the *Os internum*. If the *Funis* is attached to the middle of the *Placenta*, and that part preſents to the *Os internum* or *externum*, the whole maſs will be too bulky to come along in that poſition:

in

in this caſe you muſt introduce two fingers within the *Os externum*, and bring it down with its edge foremoſt.

When the *Placenta* is ſeparated by the contraction of the *Uterus*, in conſequence of its weight and bulk, it is puſhed down before the membranes, and both are brought away inverted.

When part of the *Placenta* hath paſſed the *Os internum*, and the reſt of it cannot be brought along by eaſy pulling, becauſe the *Os uteri* is cloſe contracted round the middle of it, or part of it ſtill adheres to the womb, ſlide the flat of your hand below the *Placenta*, through the *Os internum*; and having dilated the *Uterus*, ſlip down your hand to the edge of the cake and bring it along: but if it adheres to the *Uterus*, puſh up your hand again, and having ſeparated it cautiouſly, deliver it as before.

If inſtead of finding the edge or middle of the *Placenta* preſenting to the *Os externum* or *internum* you feel the mouth of the womb cloſely contracted, you muſt take hold of the navel-ſtring as above directed, and ſlide your other hand along the *Funis* into

into the *Vagina*; then ſlowly puſh your fingers and thumb, joined in form of a cone, through the *Os uteri*, along the ſame cord, to the place of its inſertion in the *Placenta*: here let your hand reſt, and feel with your fingers to what part of the *Uterus* the cake adheres; if it be looſe at the lower edge, try to bring it along; but if it adheres, begin and ſeparate it ſlowly, the back of your hand being turned to the *Uterus*, and the fore part of your fingers towards the *Placenta*: and for this operation the nails ought to be cut ſhort and ſmooth. In ſeparating preſs the ends of your fingers more againſt the *Placenta* than the *Uterus*, and if you cannot diſtinguiſh which is which, becauſe both feel ſoft (though the *Uterus* is firmer than the *Placenta*, and this laſt more ſolid than coagulated blood) I ſay, in this caſe ſlide down your fingers to its edge, and conduct them by the ſeparated part, preſſing it gently from the *Uterus*, until the whole is diſengaged. Sometimes, when part of it is ſeparated, the reſt will looſen and come along if you pull gently at the detached portion; but if this is not effected with eaſe, let the

whole

whole of it be ſeparated in the moſt cautious manner: ſometimes, alſo, by graſping the inſide of the *Placenta* with your hand, the whole will be looſened without further trouble. As the *Placenta* comes along, ſlide down your hand and take hold of the lower edge, by which it muſt be extracted, becauſe it is too bulky to be brought away altogether in a heap; and let it be delivered as whole as poſſible, keeping your thumb or fingers fixed upon the navel-ſtring, by which means laceration is often prevented.

When the woman lies on her back, and the *Placenta* adheres to the left ſide of the *Uterus*, it will be moſt commodious to ſeparate the cake with the right hand; whereas the left hand is moſt conveniently uſed when the *Placenta* adheres to the right ſide of the womb: but when it is attached to the forepart, back, or *Fundus*, either hand will anſwer the purpoſe.

That part of the *Uterus* to which the *Placenta* adheres, is kept ſtill diſtended, while all the reſt of it is contracted.

The nearer the adheſion is to the *Os internum*, the eaſier is the *Placenta* ſeparated, and

and *vice verſa*; becauſe it is difficult to reach up to the *Fundus*, on account of the contraction of the *Os internum* and lower part of the womb, which are not ſtretched again without great force, after they have been contracted for any length of time.

When, therefore, the *Placenta* adheres to the *Fundus*, and all the lower part of the womb is ſtrongly contracted, the hand muſt be forced up in form of a cone into the *Vagina*, and then gradually dilate the *Os internum* and inferior part of the *Uterus*. If great force is required, exert it ſlowly, reſting between whiles, that the hand may not be cramped, nor the *Vagina* in danger of being tore from the womb; for in this caſe the *Vagina* will lengthen conſiderably upwards.

While you are thus employed, let an aſſiſtant preſs with both hands on the woman's belly; or while you puſh with one hand, preſs with the other, in order to keep down the *Uterus*, elſe it will riſe high up, and roll about like a large ball, below the lax parietes of the *Abdomen*; ſo as to hinder you from effecting the neceſſary dilatation.

When

When you have overcome this contraction, and introduced your hand into the *Fundus*, ſeparate and bring the *Placenta* along, as above directed; and ſhould the *Uterus* be contracted in the middle like an hour-glaſs, a circumſtance that ſometimes, though rarely happens, the ſame method muſt be practiſed.

In every caſe, and eſpecially when the *Placenta* hath been delivered with difficulty, introduce your hand after its extraction, in order to examine if any part of the *Uterus* be pulled down and inverted; and if that be the caſe, puſh it up and reduce it without loſs of time, then clear it of the coagulated blood, which otherwiſe may occaſion violent after-pains.

For the moſt part, in ten, fifteen, or twenty minutes, more or leſs, the *Placenta* will come away of itſelf; and though ſome portion of it, or of the membranes, be left in the *Uterus*, provided no great flooding enſues, it is commonly diſcharged in a day or two, without any detriment to the woman: but at any rate, if poſſible, all the ſecundines ought to be extracted at once, and be-

fore

fore you leave your patient, in order to avoid reflections.

I find that both amongſt the ancients and moderns there have been different opinions and directions about delivering the *Placenta*; ſome alledging, that it ſhould be delivered ſlowly, or left to come of itſelf; others, that the hand ſhould be immediately introduced into the *Uterus*, to ſeparate and bring it away. Before we run into extremes of either ſide, it ſhould be conſidered how nature of herſelf acts in theſe caſes: we find in the common courſe of labours, that not once in fifty or an hundred times there is any thing more to be done than to receive the child. Some of the ancients have alledged, that no danger happens on this account oftner than once in one thouſand labours; and as nature is, for the moſt part, ſufficient of itſelf in ſuch caſes, it is very rare, perhaps not once in twenty or thirty times, that I have occaſion to ſeparate, as it generally comes down by the common aſſiſtance of pulling gently at the *Funis*, and the efforts of the woman: I alſo find, that the mouth of the womb is as eaſily dilated ſome hours after delivery, as at any other time; ſo in my opinion we ought to go in the middle way, never to aſſiſt but when we find it neceſſary: on the one hand, not to torture nature when it is ſelf-ſufficient, nor delay too long, becauſe it is poſſible that the *Placenta* ſhould be ſometimes, though ſeldom, retained ſeveral days; and if the *Uterus* ſhould be inflamed from any accident, and the woman be loſt, the operator will be blamed for leaving the after-birth behind.

CHAP. III.

Of Laborious Labours.

SECT. I.

How Laborious Labours *are occaſioned.*

IN the foregoing ſheets, which treat of natural labours, I have deſcribed the moſt eaſy and ſimple method of managing the woman, delivering the child, and extracting the *Placenta*; but as it ſometimes happens, that we muſt uſe extraordinary aſſiſtance for the preſervation of the woman or child, or both,

I muſt proceed to give directions how to behave in the laborious births, which more frequently occur than the præternatural.

A general outcry hath been raiſed againſt gentlemen of the profeſſion, as if they delighted in uſing inſtruments and violent methods in the courſe of their practice; and this clamour hath proceeded from the ignorance of ſuch as do not know that inſtruments are ſometimes abſolutely neceſſary, or from the intereſted views of ſome low, obſcure, and illiterate practitioners, both male and female, who think they find their account in decrying the practice of their neighbours. It is not to be denied, that miſchief has been done by inſtruments in the hands of the unſkilful and unwary, but I am perſuaded, that every judicious practitioner will do every thing for the ſafety of his patients before he has recourſe to any violent method, either with the hand or inſtrument; though caſes will occur, in which gentle methods will abſolutely fail. It is therefore neceſſary to explain thoſe reinforcements which muſt be uſed in dangerous labours; though they ought by no means to be called in, except when the life of the mother or child, or both, is evidently at ſtake; and even then managed with the utmoſt caution: for my own part, I have always avoided them as far as I thought conſiſtent with the ſafety of my patients, and ſtrongly inculcated the ſame maxim upon thoſe who have ſubmitted to my inſtructions.

All thoſe caſes in which the head of the child preſents, and cannot be delivered in the natural way deſcribed in chap. 2, ſect. 2. of this book, are accounted more or leſs laborious, according to the different circumſtances from which the difficulty ariſes; and theſe commonly are, firſt, Great weakneſs, proceeding from loſs of appetite and bad digeſtion; frequent vomitings, diarrhœas or dyſenteries, floodings, or any other diſeaſe that may exhauſt the patient; as alſo the fatigue ſhe may have undergone by unſkilful treatment in the beginning of labour.

Secondly, From exceſſive grief and anxiety of mind, occaſioned by the unſeaſonable news of ſudden misfortune in time of labour; which often affect her ſo, as to carry

off

off the pains, and endanger her ſinking under the ſhock.

Thirdly, From the rigidity of the *Os uteri*, *Vagina*, and external parts, which commonly happens to women in the firſt birth, eſpecially to thoſe who are about the age of forty: though it may be alſo owing to large calloſities, produced from laceration or ulceration of the parts; or to glands and ſchirrous tumours that block up the *Vagina*.

Fourthly, From a too ſmall or diſtorted *Pelvis*, which often occurs in very little women, or ſuch as have been ricketty in their childhood.

Fifthly, From the extraordinary oſſification of the child's head, by which the bones of the ſkull are hindered from yielding, as they are forced into the *Pelvis*; and from a *Hydrocephalus* or dropſy, diſtending the head to ſuch a degree, that it cannot paſs along until the water is diſcharged.

Sixthly, From the wrong preſentation of the child's head; that is, when the forehead is towards the groin or middle of the *Os pubis*; when the face preſents with the chin to the *Pubis*, *Iſchium*, or *Sacrum*; when the

 crown

crown of the head reſts above the *Os pubis*, and the forehead or face is preſſed into the hollow of the *Sacrum*; and laſtly, when one of the ears preſents.

Seventhly, When the under-part of the *Uterus* is contracted before the ſhoulders, or the body intangled in the navel-ſtring.

In all theſe caſes, except when the *Pelvis* is too narrow and the head too large, provided the head lies at the upper-part of the brim, or (though preſſed into the *Pelvis*) can be eaſily puſhed back into the *Uterus*, the beſt method is, to turn the child and deliver by the feet, according to the directions which ſhall be given in the ſequel: but if the head is preſſed into the middle or lower part of the *Pelvis*, and the *Uterus* ſtrongly contracted round the child, delivery ought to be performed with the forceps; and in all the ſeven caſes, if the woman is in danger, and if you can neither turn nor deliver with the forceps, the head muſt be opened and delivered with the crotchets. Laborious caſes from ſome of the above recited cauſes, happen much oftner than thoſe we call præternatural; but thoſe which proceed from a

nar-

narrow *Pelvis*, or a large head, are of the worſt conſequence. Theſe caſes demand greater judgment in the operator than thoſe in which the child's head does not preſent; becauſe in theſe laſt we know, that the beſt and ſafeſt method is to deliver by the feet; whereas in laborious births, we muſt maturely conſider the cauſe that retards the head from coming along, together with the neceſſary aſſiſtance required; we muſt determine when we ought to wait patiently for the efforts of nature, and when it is abſolutely neceſſary to come to her aid. If we attempt to ſuccour her too ſoon, and uſe much force in the operation, ſo that the child and mother, or one of the two, are loſt, we will be apt to reproach ourſelves for having acted prematurely, upon the ſuppoſition, that if we had waited a little longer, the pains might have, by degrees, delivered the child; or at leaſt forced the head ſo low, as that we might have extracted it with more ſafety by the aſſiſtance of the forceps. On the other hand, when we leave it to nature, perhaps by the ſtrong preſſure upon the head and brain, the child is dead when delivered, and the woman ſo exhauſted with tedious labour, that her life is in imminent danger: in this caſe, we blame ourſelves for delaying our help ſo long, reflecting, that had we delivered the patient ſooner, without paying ſuch ſcrupulous regard to the life of the child, the woman might have recovered without having run ſuch a dangerous riſk. Doubtleſs it is our duty to ſave both mother and child, if poſſible; but if that is impracticable, to pay our chief regard to the parent: and in all dubious caſes, to act cautiouſly and circumſpectly, to the beſt of our judgment and ſkill.

If the head is advanced into the *Pelvis*, and the *Uterus* ſtrongly contracted round the child, great force is required to puſh it back into the womb, becauſe the effort muſt be ſufficient to ſtretch the *Uterus*, ſo as to readmit the head, together with your hand and arm; and even then the child will be turned with great difficulty.

Should you turn when the head is too large, you may bring down the body of the child, but the head will ſtick faſt above, and cannot be extracted without the help of the crot-

crotchets; yet the caſe is ſtill worſe in a narrow *Pelvis*, even though the head be of an ordinary ſize. When things are ſo ſituated, you ſhould not attempt to turn, becauſe in ſo doing you may give the woman a great deal of pain, and yourſelf much unneceſſary fatigue: you ought, therefore, to try the forceps, and if they do not ſucceed, diminiſh the ſize of the head, and extract it, as ſhall be afterwards ſhewn.

SECT. II.

Of the FILLETS *and* FORCEPS.

WE have already obſerved, that the greateſt number of difficult and lingering labours proceed from the head's ſticking faſt in the *Pelvis*, which ſituation is occaſioned by one of the ſeven cauſes recited above: when formerly this was the caſe, the child was generally loſt, unleſs it could be turned and delivered by the feet; or if it could be extracted alive, either died ſoon after delivery, or recovered with great difficulty from the long and ſevere compreſſion of the head, while the life of the mother was endangered from the ſame cauſe as above deſcribed: for the preſſure being reciprocal, the fibres and veſſels of the ſoft parts contained in the *Pelvis* are bruiſed by the child's head, and the circulation of the fluids obſtructed; ſo that a violent inflammation, and ſometimes a ſudden mortification, enſues. If the child could not be turned, the method practiſed in theſe caſes was, to open the head and extract with the crotchet; and this expedient produced a general clamour among the women, who obſerved, that when recourſe was had to the aſſiſtance of a man-midwife, either the mother or child, or both, were loſt. This cenſure, which could not fail of being a great diſcouragement to male practitioners, ſtimulated the ingenuity of ſeveral gentlemen of the profeſſion, in order to contrive ſome gentler method of bringing along the head, ſo as to ſave the child, without any prejudice to the mother.

Their endeavours have not been without ſucceſs: a more ſafe and certain expedient for this purpoſe hath been invented, and of late brought to greater perfection in this than in any other kingdom; ſo that if we are called

called in before the child is dead, or the parts of the woman in danger of a mortification, both the *Fœtus* and mother may frequently be happily ſaved. This fortunate contrivance is no other than the forceps, which was, as is alledged, firſt uſed here by the *Chamberlains*; by whom it was kept as a noſtrum, and after their deceaſe ſo imperfectly known, as to be ſeldom applied with ſucceſs: ſo that different practitioners had recourſe to different kinds of fillets or lacks. Blunt hooks alſo, of various make, covered with leather, were invented in *England*, *France*, and other parts. The forceps, ſince the time of Dr. *Chamberlain*, have undergone ſeveral alterations, particularly in the joining, handles, form, and compoſition.

The common way of uſing them formerly, was by introducing each blade at random, taking hold of the head any how, pulling it ſtraight along, and delivering with downright force and violence; by which means, both *Os internum* and *Externum* were often tore, and the child's head much bruiſed.

On

On account of theſe bad conſequences, they had been altogether diſuſed by many practitioners, ſome of whom endeavoured, in lieu of them, to introduce divers kinds of fillets over the child's head; but none of them can be ſo eaſily uſed, or have near ſo many advantages as the forceps, when rightly applied and conducted, according to the directions that ſhall be laid down in the next ſection.

Mr. *Chapman*, as mentioned in the introduction, was the firſt author who deſcribed the forceps, with the method of uſing them; and we find in the obſervations of *Giffard*, ſeveral caſes in which he delivered and ſaved the child by the aſſiſtance of this inſtrument. A forceps was alſo contrived at *Paris*, a drawing of which may be ſeen in the medical eſſays of *Edinburgh*, in a paper communicated by Mr. *Butter*, ſurgeon: but after Mr. *Chapman* had publiſhed a delineation of his inſtrument, which was that originally uſed by the *Chamberlains*, the *French* adopted the ſame ſpecies, which among them went under the denomination of *Chapman*'s forceps. For my own part, finding in practice, that by the directions of *Chapman*, *Giffard*, and *Gregoire* at *Paris*, I frequently could not move the head along without contusing it, and tearing the parts of the woman; for they direct us to introduce the blades of the forceps where they will easiest pass, and taking hold of the head in any part of it, to extract with more or less force, according to the resistance: I therefore, (having before converted my principal attention to the study of Midwifery) began to consider the whole in a mechanical view, and reduce the extraction of the child to the rules of moving bodies in different directions: in consequence of this plan, I more accurately surveyed the dimensions and form of the *Pelvis*, together with the figure of the child's head, and the manner in which it passed along in natural labours; and from the knowledge of these things, I not only delivered with greater ease and safety than before, but also had the satisfaction to find, in teaching, that I could convey a more distinct idea of the art in this mechanical light than in any other; and particularly, gave more sure and solid directions for applying the forceps, even to the

con-

conviction of many old practitioners, when they reflected on the uncertainty attending the old method of application. From this knowledge, too, joined with experience and hints which have occurred and been communicated to me, in the course of teaching and practice, I have been led to alter the form and dimensions of the forceps, [as now made by Mr. *Best*, in *Lombard-Street*] so as to avoid the inconveniencies that attended the use of the former kinds.

The consideration of mechanicks applied to Midwifery, is likeways in no case more useful than when the child must be turned and delivered by the feet; because, there we are principally to regard the contraction of the *Uterus*, the position of the child, and the method of moving a body confined in such a manner: but I have advanced nothing in mechanics, but what I find useful in practice, and in conveying a distinct notion of the several difficulties that occur, to those who are or have been under my instruction, for whom this treatise is principally designed.

The lacks or fillets are of different kinds, of which the most simple is a noose made

on

on the end of a fillet or limber garter: but this can only be applied, before the head is faſt jammed in the *Pelvis*, or when it can be puſhed up and raiſed above the brim. The *Os externum* and *internum* having been gradually dilated, this nooſe muſt be conveyed on the ends of the fingers, and ſlipped over the fore and hind head. There are alſo other kinds differently introduced upon various blunt inſtruments, too tedious either to deſcribe or uſe: but the moſt uſeful of all theſe contrivances, is a fillet made in form of a ſheath, mounted upon a piece of ſlender whale-bone, about two feet in length, which is eaſier applied than any other expedient of the ſame kind.

When the head is high up in the *Pelvis*, if the woman has been long in labour, and the waters diſcharged for a conſiderable time, the *Uterus* being ſtrongly contracted, ſo as that the head and ſhoulders cannot be raiſed or the child turned to be delivered by the feet, while the mother is enfeebled and the pains ſo weak, that unleſs aſſiſted, ſhe is in danger of her life; alſo when the *Os internum*, *Vagina*, and *Labia Pudendi* are inflamed and

tume-

tumefied; or when there is a violent discharge of blood from the *Uterus*, provided the *Pelvis* is not too narrow, nor the head too large, this fillet may be ſucceſsfully uſed; in which caſe, if the *Os externum* and *internum* are not already ſufficiently open, they muſt be gradually dilated as much as poſſible, by the hand, which at the ſame time muſt be introduced and paſſed along the ſide of the head, in order to aſcertain the poſition thereof. This being known, let the other hand introduce the double of the whale-bone and fillet over the face and chin, where you can have the beſt purchaſe, and where it will be leaſt apt to ſlip and loſe its hold. This application being effected, let the hand be brought down, and the whole bone drawn from the ſheath of the fillet, which (after the ends of it are tied together) muſt be pulled during every pain, preſſing at the ſame time with the other hand, upon the oppoſite part of the head, and uſing more or leſs force, according to the reſiſtance.

The diſadvantage attending all fillets, is the difficulty in introducing and fixing them; and though this laſt is eaſier applied than the others,

others, yet when the *Vertix* preſents, the child's chin is ſo preſſed to the breaſt, that it is often impracticable to inſinuate the fillet between them, and if it is fixed upon the face or hind head, it frequently ſlips off in pulling: but, granting it commodiouſly fixed, when the head is large or the *Pelvis* narrow, ſo that we are obliged to pull with great force, the fillet will gall, and even cut the ſoft parts to the very bone, and if the child comes out of a ſudden, in conſequence of violent pulling, the external parts of the woman, are in great danger of ſudden laceration; but, if the head is ſmall, and comes along with a moderate force, the child may be delivered by this contrivance, without any bad conſequence: though in this caſe, we find by experience, that unleſs the woman has ſome very dangerous ſymptom, the head will in time, ſlide gradually down into the *Pelvis*, even when it is too large to be extracted with the fillet or forceps, and the child be ſafely delivered by the labour-pains, although ſlow and lingering, and the mother ſeems weak and exhauſted, provided ſhe be ſupported with nouriſhing and ſtrengthening cordials.

From

From what I have ſaid, the reader ought not to imagine, that I am more bigotted to any one contrivance than to another: as my chief ſtudy hath been to improve the art of Midwifery, I have conſidered a great many different methods, with a view of fixing upon that which ſhould beſt ſucceed in practice: I have tried ſeveral kinds of lacks, which have been from time to time recommended to me, and in particular, the laſt mentioned fillet, which was communicated to me by the learned Doctor MEAD nine years ago. As this fillet could in all appearance, be more eaſily introduced than any other, I, for ſeveral years, carried it with me, when I was called in difficult caſes, and frequently uſed it accordingly; but, I generally found the fixing of this, as well as all other lacks, ſo uncertain, that I was obliged to have recourſe to the forceps, which being introduced with greater eaſe, and fixed with more certainty, ſeldom failed to anſwer the purpoſe, better than any other method hitherto found out: but, let not this aſſertion prevent people of ingenuity from employing their talents in improving theſe or any other methods that may be ſafe and uſeful: for daily experience

proves

proves, that we are ſtill imperfect and very far from the *Ne plus Ultra* of diſcovery in arts and ſciences: though I hope every gentleman will deſpiſe and avoid the character of a ſelfiſh ſecret-monger.

As the head is forced along the *Pelvis*, commonly in theſe laborious caſes the bones of the *Cranium* are ſo compreſſed, that they ride over one another, ſo that the bulk of the whole is diminiſhed, and the head as it is puſhed forward, is from a round, altered into an oblong figure: when therefore it is advanced into the *Pelvis*, where it ſticks faſt for a conſiderable time, and cannot be delivered by the labour pains, the forceps may be introduced with great eaſe and ſafety, like a pair of artificial hands, by which the head is very little (if at all) mark'd, and the woman very ſeldom tore. But, if the head is detained above the brim of the *Pelvis*, or a ſmall portion of it only farther advanced, and it appears, that the one being too narrow, or the other too large, the woman cannot be delivered by the ſtrongeſt labour pains; in that caſe, the child cannot be ſaved, either by turning and bringing it by the feet, or delivered by the application of fillet or forceps;

ceps; but the operator muſt unavoidably uſe the diſagreeable method of extracting with the crotchet. Nevertheleſs, in all theſe caſes, the forceps ought firſt to be tried, and ſometimes they will ſucceed beyond expectation, provided the birth is retarded by the weakneſs of the woman, and the ſecond, third, ſixth, or ſeventh obſtructions: but they cannot be depended upon, even when the *Vertex* preſents, with the forehead to the ſide or back part of the *Pelvis*, and (tho' the woman has had ſtrong pains for many hours after the membranes are broke) the head is not forced down into the *Pelvis*, or at leaſt, but an inconſiderable part of it, reſembling the ſmall end of a ſugar loaf. For, from theſe circumſtances, you may conclude, that the largeſt part of it is ſtill above the brim, and that either the head is too large, or the *Pelvis* too narrow. Even in theſe caſes, indeed, the laſt fillet or a long pair of forceps may take ſuch a firm hold, that with great force and the ſtrong purchaſe, the head will be delivered: but ſuch violence is commonly fatal to the woman, by cauſing ſuch an inflammation, and perhaps laceration of the parts, as is attended with mortification. In order to diſable young practitioners from running ſuch

ſuch riſks, and to free myſelf from the temptation of uſing too great force, I have always uſed and recommended the forceps ſo ſhort in the handles, that they cannot be uſed with ſuch violence as will endanger the woman's life; though the purchaſe of them is ſufficient to extract the head, when one half or two thirds of it are equal to, or paſt the upper or narrow part of the *Pelvis*.

When the head is high, the forceps may be locked in the middle of the *Pelvis*; but in that caſe, great care muſt be taken in feeling with the fingers all round, that no part of the *Vagina* be included in the locking. Sometimes, when the head reſts, or is preſſed too much on the forepart or ſide of the *Pelvis*, either at the brim or lower down, by introducing one blade, it may be moved farther down, provided the labour-pains are ſtrong, and the operation aſſiſted by the fingers of the other hand applied to the oppoſite ſide of the head; but if the fingers cannot reach high enough, the beſt method is to turn or move the blade towards the ear of the child, and introduce the other along the oppoſite ſide.

In a narrow *Pelvis* I have ſometimes found the head of the child thrown ſo much forward over the *Os pubis*, by the jetting in of the *Sacrum* and lower *Vertebra* of the loins, that I could not puſh the handles of the forceps far enough back, to include, within the blades, the bulky part of the head which lay over the *Pubis*. To remedy this inconvenience, I contrived a longer pair, curved on one ſide, and convex on the other: but theſe ought never to be uſed except when the head is ſmall; for, as we have already obſerved, when the head is large, and the greateſt part of it remains above the brim, the parts of the woman may be inflamed and contuſed by the exertion of too much force. Neverthleleſs, this kind of forceps may be advantageouſly uſed when the face preſents and is low down, and the chin turned to the *Sacrum*; becauſe in that caſe, the *Occiput* is towards the *Pubis*, ſo that the ends of the blades can take firmer hold of the head; but then the chin cannot be turned below the *Pubis* ſo eaſily with theſe as with the other kind, when the hindhead cannot be brought below theſe laſt bones.

SECT.

SECT. III.

General rules for uſing the FORCEPS.

THE farther the head is advanced in the *Pelvis*, the eaſier is it delivered with the forceps; becauſe then it is changed from a round to an oblong figure, by being forced along by the labour-pains: on the contrary, when the head remains high up, reſting upon the brim of the *Pelvis*, the forceps are uſed with greater difficulty and uncertainty.

The *Os externum* muſt be gradually opened by introducing the fingers one after another, in form of a cone, after they have been lubricated with pomatum, moving and turning them in a ſemicircular motion, as they are puſhed up. If the head is ſo low down that the hand cannot be introduced high up in this form, let the parts be dilated by the fingers turned in the direction of the *Coccyx*, the back of the hand being upwards next to the child's head: the external parts being ſufficiently opened to admit all the fingers, let the back of the hand be turned to the *Perineum*, while the fingers and thumb being flattened, will ſlide along betwixt the head and the *Os ſacrum*. If the right hand be uſed, let it be turned a little to the left ſide of the *Pelvis*, becauſe the broad ligament and membrane that fill up the ſpace between the *Sacrum* and *Iſchia*, will yield and allow more room for the fingers to advance; for the ſame reaſon, when the left hand is introduced, it muſt be turned a little to the right ſide. Having gained your point ſo far, continue to puſh up until your fingers paſs the *Os internum*; at the ſame time, with the palm of your hand, raiſe or ſcoop up the head, by which means you will be more at liberty to reach higher, dilate the internal parts, and diſtinguiſh the ſituation and ſize of the head, together with the dimenſions of the *Pelvis*: from which inveſtigation you will be able to judge, whether the child ought to be turned and brought by the feet, or delivered with the forceps; or if the labour-pains are ſtrong, and the head preſents tolerably fair, without being jammed in the *Pelvis*, you will reſolve to wait ſome time, in hope of ſeeing the child delivered by the labour-pains, eſpecially when the woman is in no immediate danger, and the chief obſtacle is the rigidity of the parts.

The poſition of the head is diſtinguiſhed by feeling for one of the ears, the fore or ſmooth part of which, is towards the face of the child; if it cannot be aſcertained by this mark, the hand and fingers muſt be puſhed farther up, to feel for the face or back part of the neck; but if the head cannot be traced, the obſervation muſt be taken from the *Fontanelle*, or that part of the *Cranium* where the lambdoidal croſſes the end of the *Sagittal ſuture*. When the ears of the child are towards the ſides of the *Pelvis*, or diagonal, the forehead being either to the *Sacrum* or *Pubis*, the patient muſt lie on her back, with her breech a little over the bed, her legs and thighs being ſupported as in chap. 2. ſect. 1. and chap. 4. ſect. 4. If one ear is to the *Sacrum* and the other to the *Pubis*, ſhe muſt be laid on one ſide, with her breech over the bed as before, her knees being pulled up to her belly, and a pillow placed between them; except when the upper part of the *Sacrum* jetts too much forward, in which caſe ſhe muſt lie upon her back, as above deſcribed.

The blades of the forceps ought always, if poſſible, to be introduced along the ears; by which means they approach nearer to each other, gain a firmer hold, and hurt the head leſs than in any other direction: frequently, indeed, not the leaſt mark of their application is to be perceived; whereas, if the blades are applied along the forehead and *Occiput*, they are at a greater diſtance from each other, require more room, frequently at their points preſs in the bones of the ſkull, and endanger a laceration in the *Os externum* of the woman.

The woman being laid in a right poſition for the application of the forceps, the blades ought to be privately conveyed between the feather-bed and the cloaths, at a ſmall diſtance from one another, or on each ſide of the patient: that this conveyance may be the more eaſily effected, the legs of the inſtrument ought to be kept in the operator's ſide-pockets. Thus provided, when he ſits down to deliver, let him ſpread the ſheet that hangs over the bed upon his lap, and under that cover take out and diſpoſe the blades on each ſide of the patient; by which means, he he will often be able to deliver with the forceps, without their being perceived by the woman herſelf, or any other of the aſſiſtants. Some people pin a ſheet to each ſhoulder, and throw the other end over the bed, that they may be the more effectually concealed from the view of thoſe who are preſent: but this method is apt to confine and embarraſs the operator. At any rate, as women are commonly frightened at the very name of an inſtrument, it is adviſeable to conceal them as much as poſſible, until the character of the operator is fully eſtabliſhed.

SECT. IV.

The different ways of uſing the FORCEPS.

NUMB. I.

When the Head is down to the Os externum.

WHEN the head preſents fair, with the forehead to the *Sacrum*, the *Occiput* to the *Pubis*, and the ears to the ſides of the *Pelvis*, or a little diagonal; in this caſe, the head is commonly pretty well advanced in the baſin, and the operator ſeldom miſcarries in in the uſe of the forceps. Things being thus ſituated, let the patient be laid on her back, her head and ſhoulders being ſomewhat raiſed, and the breech advanced a little over the ſide or foot of the bed; while the aſſiſtants ſitting on each ſide ſupport her legs, at the ſame time keeping her knees duly ſeparated and raiſed up to the belly, and her lower parts always covered with the bed-cloaths, that ſhe may not be apt to catch cold. In order to avoid this inconvenience, if the bed is at a great diſtance from the fire, the weather cold, and the woman of a delicate conſtitution, a chafing-diſh with charcoal, or a veſſel with warm water, ſhould be placed near or under the bed. Theſe precautions being taken, let the operator place himſelf upon a low chair, and having lubricated with pomatum the blades of the forceps, and alſo his right hand and fingers, ſlide firſt the hand gently into the *Vagina*, puſhing it along in a flattened form, between that and the child's head, until the fingers have paſſed the *Os internum*; then, with his other hand, let him take one of the blades of the forceps from the place where it was depoſited, and intro-

duce

duce it betwixt his right hand and the head; if the point or extremity of it ſhould ſtick at the ear, let it be ſlipt backward a little, and then guided forwards with a ſlow and delicate motion: when it ſhall have paſſed the *Os uteri*, let it be advanced ſtill farther up, until the reſt at which the blades lock into each other be cloſe to the lower part of the head, or at leaſt within an inch thereof.

Having in this manner introduced one blade, let him withdraw his right hand, and inſinuate his left in the ſame direction along the other ſide of the head, until his fingers ſhall have paſſed the *Os internum*; then taking out the other blade from the place of concealment with the hand that is diſengaged, let it be applied to the other ſide of the child's head, by the ſame means employed in introducing the firſt: then the left hand muſt be withdrawn, and the head being embraced between the blades, let them be locked in each other, and the handles firmly faſtened together with a fillet or garter. Having thus ſecured them, he muſt take a firm hold with both hands, and when the pain comes on, begin to pull the head along from ſide to side, continuing this operation during every pain, until the *Vertix* appears through the *Os externum*, and the neck of the child can be felt with the finger below the *Os pubis*; at which time the forehead pushes out the *Perineum* like a large tumour: then let him stand up, and raising the handles of the forceps, pull the head upwards also, that the forehead being turned half round upwards, the *Perineum* and lower parts of the *Os externum* may not be tore.

In stretching the *Os externum* or *internum* we ought to imitate nature; for in practice we find, that when they are opened slowly, and at intervals, by the membranes with the waters, or the child's head, the parts are seldom inflamed or lacerated: but in all natural labours, when these parts are suddenly opened, and the child delivered by strong and violent pains, without much intermission, this misfortune commonly happens, and the woman is afterwards in great pain and danger.

We ought, therefore, when obliged to dilate those parts, to proceed in that slow, deliberate manner; and though upon the first trial

trial they feel ſo rigid, that one would imagine they could never yield or extend; yet by ſtretching with the hand, and reſting by intervals, we can overcome the greateſt reſiſtance. We muſt alſo, in ſuch caſes, be very cautious, pulling ſlowly, with intermiſſions, in order to prevent the ſame laceration: for which purpoſe too, we ought to lubricate the *Perineum* with pomatum, during thoſe ſhort intervals, and keep the palm of one hand cloſe preſs'd to it and the neighbouring parts, while with the other we pull at the extremity of the handles of the forceps; by which means, we preſerve the parts, and know how much we may venture to pull at a time. When the head is almoſt delivered, the parts thus ſtretched muſt be ſlipped over the forehead and face of the child, while the operator pulls upwards with the other hand, turning the handles of the forceps to the body of the woman. This method of pulling upwards raiſes the child's head from the *Perineum*, and the half-round turn to the *Abdomen* of the mother brings out the forehead and face from below: for, when that part of the hindhead which is joined to the neck,

neck, refts at the under-part of the *Pubis*, the head turns upon it as upon an axis. In præternatural cafes alfo, the body being delivered, muft in the fame manner be raifed up over the belly of the mother; and at the fame time, the *Perineum* flipt over the face and forehead of the child.

In the introduction of the forceps, let each blade be pufhed up in an imaginary line from the *Os externum*, to the middle fpace betwixt the navel and *Scrobiculum cordis* of the woman; or in other words, held as far back as the *Perineum* will allow. The introduction of the other hand to the oppofite fide, will, by preffing the child's head againft the firft blade, detain it in its proper place till the other can be applied; or if this preffure fhould not feem fufficient, it may be fupported by the operator's knee.

NUMB. II.

When higher in the Pelvis.

WHEN the head prefents, but remains very high, the forehead being at or above the upper-part of the *Sacrum*, and on account of the narrownefs of the *Pelvis* at that part, can-

cannot be brought along at the firſt or ſecond trial, let the operator turn the forehead a little on one ſide; but if it is ſo fixed in the *Pelvis* as not to be moved in that manner, let him try to puſh the head above the brim with the forceps, and then turn it to one ſide, in order to profit by the width of the baſin, which in this place is commonly about one inch greater from ſide to ſide, than from the fore to the back-part: this being done, let him pull along, until the head arrives at the lower part of the *Pelvis*, then turn the forehead into the hollow of the *Sacrum*, and the *Vertix* in below the *Os pubis*, and deliver with an half-round turn as above directed.

When the head is come low down, and cannot be brought farther, becauſe one of the ſhoulders reſts above the *Pubis*, and the other upon the upper-part of the *Sacrum*, let the head be ſtrongly graſped with the forceps, and puſhed up as far as poſſible, moving from blade to blade as you puſh up, that the ſhoulders may be the more eaſily moved to the ſides of the *Pelvis*, by turning the face or forehead a little towards one of them; then the forehead muſt be brought

back

back again into the hollow of the *Sacrum*, and another effort made to deliver: but ſhould the difficulty remain, let the head be puſhed up again, and turned to the other ſide; becauſe it is uncertain which of the ſhoulders reſts on the *Pubis* or *Sacrum:* ſuppoſe, for example, the right ſhoulder of the child ſticks above the *Pubis*, the forehead being in the hollow of the *Sacrum*; in this caſe, if the forehead be turned to the right hand ſide of the woman, the ſhoulder will not move; whereas if it be turned to the left, and the head at the ſame time puſhed a little upwards, ſo as to raiſe and diſengage the parts that were fixed, the right ſhoulder being towards the right-hand ſide, and the other to the left ſide of the brim of the *Pelvis*, when the forehead is turned back again into the hollow of the *Sacrum*, the obſtacle will be removed, and the head be more eaſily delivered. This being performed, let the forceps be unlocked, and the blades diſpoſed cautiouſly under the cloaths, ſo as not to be diſcovered; then proceed to the delivery of the child, which, when the navel-ſtring is cut and tied, may be committed to the nurſe. The next care is, to wipe the blades of the forceps, ſingly, under the cloaths, ſlide them warily into your pockets, and deliver the *Placenta*.

Though the forceps are covered with leather, and appear ſo ſimple and innocent, I have given directions for concealing them, that young practitioners, before their characters are fully eſtabliſhed, may avoid the calumnies and miſrepreſentations of thoſe people who are apt to prejudice the ignorant and weak-minded againſt the uſe of any inſtrument, though never ſo neceſſary, in this profeſſion; and who, taking the advantage of unforeſeen accidents which may afterwards happen to the patient, charge the whole miſfortune to the innocent operator.

NUMB. III.

When the forehead is to the Os pubis.

WHEN the forehead, inſtead of being towards the *Sacrum*, is turned forwards to the *Pubis*, the woman muſt be laid in the ſame poſition as in the former caſe; becauſe here alſo, the ears of the child are towards the ſides of the *Pelvis*, or a little diagonally ſituated, provided the forehead is towards one of the groins. The blades of the forceps being introduced along the ears, or as near them as poſſible, according to the foregoing directions, the head muſt be puſhed up a little, and the forehead turned to one ſide of the *Pelvis*; thus let it be brought along, until the hindhead arrives at the lower part of the *Iſchium*: then the forehead muſt be turned backward into the hollow of the *Sacrum*, and even a quarter or more to the contrary ſide, in order to prevent the ſhoulders from hitching on the upper part of the *Pubis* or *Sacrum*, ſo that they may be ſtill towards the ſides of the *Pelvis*; then let the quarter turn be reverſed, and the forehead being re-placed in the hollow of the *Sacrum*, the head may be extracted as above. In performing theſe different turns, let the head be puſhed up or pulled down occaſionally, as it meets with leaſt reſiſtance. In this caſe, when the head is ſmall, it will come along as it preſents; but if large, the chin will be ſo much preſſed againſt the breaſt, that it cannot be brought up with the half-round turn, and the woman will be tore if it comes along.

NUMB.

NUMB. IV.

When it presents fair at the brim of the PELVIS.

WHEN the forehead and face of the child is turned to the side of the *Pelvis*, (in which case it is higher than in the first situation) it will be difficult, if the woman lies on her back, to introduce the forceps so as to grasp the head with a blade over each ear; because the head is often pressed so hard against the bones, in this position, that there is no room to insinuate the fingers between the ear and the *Os pubis*, so as to introduce the blades safely, on the inside of the *Os internum*, or push one of them up between the fingers and the child's head. When things are so situated, the best posture for the woman, is that of lying on one side, as formerly directed, because the bones will yield a little, and the forceps (of consequence) may be the more easily introduced.

Suppose her lying on her left side, and the forehead of the child turned to the same side of the *Pelvis*; let the fingers of the operator's right hand be introduced along the ear, between the head and the *Os pubis*, until they paſs the *Os internum:* If the head is ſo immoveably fixed in the *Pelvis*, that there is no paſſage between them, let his left hand be puſhed up between the *Sacrum* and the child's head, which being raiſed as high as poſſible, above the brim of the *Pelvis*, he will have room ſufficient for his fingers and forceps; then let him ſlide up one of the blades with the right hand, remembring to preſs the handle backwards to the *Perineum*, that the point may humour the turn of the *Sacrum* and child's head: this being effected, let him withdraw his left hand, with which he may hold the handle of the blade already introduced, while he inſinuates the fingers of his right hand at the *Os pubis*, as before directed, and puſhes up the other blade, ſlowly and gently, that he may run no riſk of hurting the *Os internum* or bladder; and here alſo keep the handle of it as far backwards as the *Perineum* will allow: when the point has paſſed the *Os internum*, let him ſlide it up farther, and join the legs by locking them together, keeping them ſtill in a line with the middle ſpace betwixt the navel

navel and *Scrobiculum cordis.* Having tied the handles as before directed, let him pull along the head, moving it from ſide to ſide, or from one ear of the child to the other; when it is ſufficiently advanced, let him move the forehead into the hollow of the *Sacrum*, and a quarter turn farther, then bring it back into the ſame cavity; but if the head will not eaſily come along, let the woman be turned on her back after the forceps have been fixed; let the hind head be pulled half round outwards from below the *Os pubis*, and the inſtrument and child managed as before.

In all thoſe caſes that require the forceps, if the head cannot be raiſed above the brim of the *Pelvis*, or the fingers introduced within the *Os internum*, to guide the points of the forceps along the ears, eſpecially at the *Pubis*, *Iſchia* or *Sacrum*; let the fingers and hand be puſhed up as far as they will go, along the open ſpace betwixt the *Sacrum* and *Iſchium*; then one of the blades may be introduced, moved to, and fixed over the ear, the ſituation of which is already known: the other hand may be introduced, and the other blade conducted in the ſame manner, on the oppoſite ſide of the *Pelvis*; but before they are locked together, care muſt be taken that they are exactly oppoſite to each other, and both ſufficiently introduced. In this caſe, if the operator finds the upper part of the *Sacrum* jetting in ſo much, that the point of the forceps cannot paſs it, let him try with his hand to turn the forehead a little backwards, ſo that one ear will be towards the groin, and the other towards the ſide of that prominence; conſequently there will be the more room for the blades to paſs along the ears: but if the forehead ſhould remain immoveable, or though moved, return to its former place, let one blade be introduced behind one ear, and its fellow before the other, in which caſe, the introduction is ſometimes more eaſily performed when the woman lies on her back, than when ſhe is laid on one ſide.

NUMB. V.

When the FACE *preſents.*

WHEN the face preſents, reſting on the upper part of the *Pelvis*, the head ought to be be pushed up to the *Fundus uteri*, the child turned and brought by the feet, according to the directions that will be given, when we come to treat of præternatural deliveries; because the hind head is turned back on the shoulders, and unless very small, cannot be pulled along with the forceps; but should it advance pretty fast in the *Pelvis*, it will be sometimes delivered alive, without any assistance. But, if it descends slowly, or after it is low down, sticks for a considerable time, the long pressure on the brain, frequently destroys the child, if not relieved in time, by turning or extracting with the forceps.

When the head is detained very high up, and no signs of its descending appear, and the operator having stretched the parts with a view to turn, discovers that the *Pelvis* is narrow, and the head large, he must not proceed with turning, because after this hath been performed, perhaps with great difficulty, the head cannot be delivered without the assistance of the crotchet. No doubt it would be a great advantage in all cases where the face or forehead presents, if we could raise the head so as to alter the bad position, and move it ſo, with our hand, as to bring the crown of the head to preſent; and indeed, this ſhould always be tried, and more eſpecially when the *Pelvis* is too narrow, or the head too large; and when we are dubious of ſaving the child by turning: but frequently this is impoſſible to be done, when the waters are evacuated, the *Uterus* ſtrongly contracted on the child, and the upper part of the head ſo ſlippery as to elude our hold; inſomuch, that even when the preſſure is not great, we ſeldom ſucceed, unleſs the head is ſmall, and then we can ſave the child by turning. If you ſucceed and the woman is ſtrong, go on as in natural labour; but, if this fails, then it will be more adviſeable to wait with patience for the deſcent of the head, ſo as that it may be delivered with the forceps; and conſequently the child may be ſaved: but if it ſtill remains in its high ſituation, and the woman is weak and exhauſted, the forceps may be tried, and ſhould they fail, recourſe muſt be had to the crotchet; becauſe the mother's life is always to be more regarded than the ſafety of the child.

When

When the face of the child is come down and sticks at the *Os externum*, the greatest part of the head is then squeezed down into the *Pelvis*, and if not speedily delivered, the child is frequently lost by the violent compression of the brain: besides, when it is so low down, it seldom can be returned on account of the great contraction of the *Uterus*. In this case, when the chin is turned towards the *Pubis*, at the lower part of that bone, the woman must be laid on her back, the forceps introduced as formerly directed in the first case, and when the chin is brought out from under the *Pubis*, the head must be pulled half round upwards; by which means, the fore and hind head will be raised from the *Perineum*, and the under part of the *Os externum* prevented from being tore.

When the chin is towards the *Sacrum*, the hindhead pressed back betwixt the shoulders, so that the face is kept from rising up below the *Pubis*, the head must be pushed up with the hand, to the upper part of the *Pelvis*, and the forceps introduced and fixed on the ears, the hindhead must be turned to one side of the *Pelvis*, while the chin is moved to the other side, and if possible, to the lower part of the *Ischium*; then the hindhead must be brought into the hollow of the *Sacrum*, with the chin below the *Pubis*, and delivered as above directed. If this cannot be done, let the operator try, with the forceps, to pull down the hindhead below the *Pubis*, and at the same time, wi h the fingers of the other hand, push the face and forehead, backwards and upwards into the hollow of the *Sacrum*. If the chin points to either side of the *Pelvis*, the woman must be laid on her side, the blades of the forceps introduced along the ears, one at the *Pubis*, and the other at the *Sacrum*; and the chin when brought lower down, turned to the *Pubis*, and delivered; for the *Pelvis* being only two inches in depth at this place, the chin is easily brought from under it, and then the head is at liberty to be turned half round upwards; because the chin being disengaged from this bone, can be pulled up over it externally; by which means, two inches of room, at least, will be gained for the more easy delivery of the fore and hindhead, which are now pressed against the *Perinæum*.

But,

But, if the chin points to the back part of the *Pelvis*, the forehead is ſqueezed againſt the *Pubis*, while the hindhead is preſſed upon the back betwixt the ſhoulders; ſo that the head cannot be delivered, unleſs the *Occiput* can be brought out from below the *Pubis*, as formerly deſcribed.

The ſum of all that has been ſaid on this head, may be comprehended in the following general maxims.

Young practitioners are often at a loſs to know and judge by the touch in the *Vagina*, when the head is far enough down in the baſin, for uſing the forceps. If we were to take our obſervations from what we feel of the head, at the *Pubis*, we ſhould be frequently deceived, becauſe in that place the *Pelvis* is only two inches in depth, and the head will ſeem lower down than it really is: but if in examining backwards, we find little or no part of it towards the *Sacrum*, we may be certain, that all the head is above the brim: if we find it down as far as the middle of the *Sacrum*, one third of it is advanced; if as far down as the lower part, one half; and in this caſe, the largeſt part is equal with the brim. When it is in this ſituation,

tuation, we may be almoſt certain of ſucceeding with the forceps; and when the head is ſo low as to protrude the external parts, they never fail. But theſe things will differ according to different circumſtances, that may occaſion a tedious delivery.

Let the operator acquire an accurate knowledge of the figure, ſhape and dimenſions of the *Pelvis*, together with the ſhape, ſize and poſition of the child's head.

Let the breech of the woman, be always brought forewards, a little over the bed, and her thighs pulled up to her belly, whether ſhe lies on her ſide or back, to give room to apply, and to move the forceps up or down, or from ſide to ſide.

Let the parts be opened and the fingers paſs the *Os internum*; in order to which, if it cannot be otherwiſe accompliſhed, let the head be raiſed two or three inches, that the fingers may have more room; if the head can be raiſed above the brim your hand is not confined by the bones: for, as we have already obſerved, the *Pelvis* is wider from ſide to ſide, at the brim, than at the lower part: if the fingers are not paſt the *Os uteri*,

it

it is in danger of being included betwixt the forceps and the child's head.

The forceps, if poſſible, ſhould paſs along the ears, becauſe, in that caſe, they ſeldom or never hurt or mark the head.

They ought to be puſhed up in an imaginary line, towards the middle ſpace between the navel and *Scrobiculum cordis*, otherwiſe, the ends will run againſt the *Sacrum*.

The forehead ought always to be turned into the hollow of the *Sacrum*, when it is not already in that ſituation.

When the face preſents, the chin muſt be turned to below the *Pubis*, and the hindhead into the hollow of the *Sacrum*.

When the ſhoulders reſt at the *Pubis*, where they are detained, the head muſt be turned a large quarter to the oppoſite ſide, ſo as that they may lie towards the ſides of the *Pelvis*.

The head muſt always be brought out with an half round turn over the outſide of the *Pubis*, for the preſervation of the *Perinæum*, which muſt, at the ſame time, be ſupported

ported with the flat of the other hand, and slid gently backwards over the head.

Almost all these directions are to be followed, except when the head is small, in which case it may be brought along by the force of pulling: but this only happens when the woman is reduced, and the labour-pains are not sufficient to deliver the child; for the lower part of the *Uterus* may be so strongly contracted before the shoulders, and so close to the neck of the child, as to prevent its advancing, even when the head is so loose in the *Pelvis*, that we can sometimes push our fingers all round it; and this is oftnest the occasion of preventing the head's being delivered when low in the *Pelvis*. The difficulty, when high up, is from the restraint at the brim, and when it passes that, the head is seldom retained in the lower part, unless the patient is weak. In this case, we need not wait, because we are commonly certain of relieving the woman immediately, with the forceps, by which you prevent the danger that may happen both to the mother and child, by the head's continuing to lodge there too long. This case should

ſhould be a caution againſt breaking the membranes too ſoon, that the *Uterus* may not contract too forcibly and too long before the ſhoulder; when the head is advanced one third or half way on the outſide of the *Os externum*, which laſt inconvenience is frequently remedied by introducing your two fingers into the *Rectum*, as formerly directed; by theſe rules, delivery may (for the moſt part) be performed with eaſe and ſafety: nevertheleſs, the head is ſometimes ſo ſqueezed and locked in the *Pelvis*, and the hairy ſcalp ſo much ſwelled, that it is impracticable to raiſe up the head, ſo as to come at the ears or *Os internum*; or to diſtinguiſh the ſutures of the ſkull, ſo as to know how the head preſents. In this caſe, the forceps muſt be introduced at random, and the uncertainty of the poſition, generally removed by remembring, that in thoſe caſes, where the head is ſqueezed down with great difficulty, the ears are for the moſt part, towards the *Pubis* and *Sacrum*; and that the forehead ſeldom turns into the hollow of the *Sacrum*, before the *Occiput* is come down to the lower part of the *Iſchium*; and then riſes gradually towards

wards the under part of the *Pubis*, and the *Perinæum* and *Anus* are forced down before it, in form of a large tumour.

On ſuch occaſions, the woman being laid on her ſide, if one ear is to the *Sacrum* and the other to the *Pubis*, the blades of the forceps are to be introduced; and if they meet with any reſiſtance at the points, they muſt not be forcibly thruſt up, leſt they paſs on the outſide of the *Os uteri*, and tear the *Vagina*, which, together with the womb, would be included in the inſtrument and pulled along with the head: for this reaſon, if the blade does not eaſily paſs, let it be withdrawn a little downwards, as before directed, and puſhed up again, moving the point cloſe to the head; if the ear obſtructs its paſſage, let the point be brought a little outwards: and by theſe cautious eſſays, it will at length paſs without further reſiſtance, and ought to be advanced a conſiderable way, in order to certify the operator that he is not on the outſide of the *Os internum*.

When the forceps are fixed, and the operator uncertain which way the forehead lies, let him pull ſlowly, and move the head with a quarter turn, firſt to one ſide and then to the other, until he ſhall have found the direction in which it comes moſt eaſily along.

If at any time we find the forceps begin to ſlip, we muſt reſt, and puſh them up again gently: but if they are like to ſlide off at a ſide, untie the handles, and move them ſo as to take a firmer hold, fix as before, and deliver. If we are obliged to hold with both hands, the parts may be ſupported by the firm application of an aſſiſtant's hand; for without ſuch cautious management, they will run a great riſk of being lacerated: a misfortune which rarely happens, when the *Perineum* is properly preſſed back, and the head leiſurely delivered. Sometimes, when the head is brought low down, you may take off the forceps, and help along with your fingers on each ſide of the *Coccyx*, or in the *Rectum*, as directed in the natural labour.

If the head is low down, the ears are commonly diagonal, or to the ſides; and when the head is brought down one third, or one half, through the *Os externum*, the operator can then certify himſelf, whether the forehead is turned to the *Coccyx* or *Pubis*, by feeling with his finger for the back-part of the neck or ear, betwixt the *Pubis* and the head; and then move the head as above directed.

Let him try to alter with his hand, every bad poſition of the head; and if it be detained high up in the *Pelvis* in conſequence of the woman's weakneſs, the rigidity of the parts, the circumvolutions or ſhortneſs of the *Funis*, or the contraction of the *Uterus* over the ſhoulders of the child, the forceps will frequently ſucceed when the *Fœtus* cannot be turned: but if the head is large, or the *Pelvis* narrow, the child is ſeldom ſaved either by turning or uſing the forceps, until the head ſhall be farther advanced. And here it will not be amiſs to obſerve, that the blades of the forceps ought to be new covered with ſtripes of waſhed leather, after they ſhall have been uſed, eſpecially in delivering a woman ſuſpected of having an infectious diſtemper.

SECT. V.

When and how to uſe the CROTCHET.

NUMB. I.

WHEN the head preſents, and cannot be delivered by the labour-pains; when all the common methods have been uſed with-

without ſucceſs, the woman being exhauſted, and all her efforts vain; and when the child cannot be delivered without ſuch force as will endanger the life of the mother, becauſe the head is too large or the *Pelvis* too narrow; it then becomes abſolutely neceſſary to open the head, and extract with the hand, forceps, or crotchet. Indeed, this laſt method formerly was the common practice when the child could not be eaſily turned, and is ſtill in uſe with thoſe who do not know how to ſave the child by delivering with the forceps: for this reaſon, their chief care and ſtudy was to diſtinguiſh, whether the *Fœtus* was dead or alive; and as the ſigns were uncertain, the operation was often delayed until the woman was in the moſt imminent danger; or when it was performed ſooner, the operator was frequently accuſed of raſhneſs, on the ſuppoſition, that the child might in time have been delivered alive by the labour-pains: perhaps he was ſometimes conſcious to himſelf of the juſtice of this imputation, although what he had done was with an upright intention.

The ſigns of a dead *Fœtus* were, firſt, the child's ceaſing to move and ſtir in the *Uterus.* Secondly, The evacuation of meconium, though the breech is not preſſed into the *Pelvis.* Thirdly, No perceiveable pulſation at the *Fontanelle* and temporal arteries. Fourthly, a large ſwelling or tumour of the hairy ſcalp. Fifthly, An uncommon laxity of the bones of the *Cranium.* Sixthly, The diſcharge of a fœtid *Ichor* from the *Vagina*, the effluvia of which ſurround the woman, and gave riſe to the opinion, that her breath conveyed a mortified ſmell. Seventhly, Want of motion in the tongue, when the face preſents. Eighthly, No perceivable pulſation in the arteries of the *Funis umbilicalis*, when it falls down below the head; nor at the wriſt when the arm preſents; and no motion of the fingers. Ninthly, The pale and livid countenance of the woman. Tenthly, A collapſing and flaccidity of the breaſts. Eleventhly, A coldneſs felt in the *Abdomen*, and weight, from the child's falling like a heavy ball to the ſide on which ſhe lies. Twelfthly, A ſeparation of the hairy ſcalp

on

on the ſlighteſt touch, and a diſtinct perception of the bare bones.

All or moſt of theſe ſigns are dubious and uncertain, except the laſt, which can only be obſerved after the *Fœtus* hath been dead ſeveral days. One may alſo certainly pronounce the child's death, if no pulſation hath been felt in the navel-ſtring for the ſpace of twenty or thirty minutes; but the ſame certainty is not to be acquired from the arm, unleſs the ſkin can be ſtripped off with eaſe.

NUMB. II.

MIDWIFERY is now ſo much improved, that the neceſſity of deſtroying the child does not occur ſo often as formerly; indeed it never ſhould be done, except when it is impoſſible to turn, or to deliver with the forceps; and this is ſeldom the caſe, but when the *Pelvis* is too narrow, or the head too large to paſs, and therefore reſts above the brim: for this reaſon it is not ſo neceſſary for the operator to puzzle himſelf about dubious ſigns; becauſe in theſe two caſes, there is no room for heſitation: for if the woman cannot poſſibly be delivered in any other way, and is in imminent danger of her life, the best practice is undoubtedly to have recourse to that method which alone can be used for her preservation, namely, To diminish the bulk of the head.

SECT. VI.

The old method of extracting the HEAD.

VARIOUS have been the contrivances intended for this purpose: some practitioners, when the head did not advance in the *Pelvis*, introduced the *Speculum matricis*, in order to stretch the bones asunder, and thereby increase the capacity of the basin; if, after this operation, the woman could not be delivered with her pains, they fixed a large screw in the head, by which they pulled with gteat force. Others opened the head with a large bistory, or a short broad-bladed knife, in form of a myrtle leaf; or with a crooked bistory, with a long handle: then a small pair of forceps with teeth were introduced, and one blade being insinuated into the opening, they laid hold on the skull, and pulled the head along. If this method failed,

failed, according to *Albucaſis*, they uſed another kind much larger, to graſp the whole head: they likewiſe made uſe of different kinds of crotchets, both ſharp and blunt; and when the head was lower down, they practiſed the ſame expedients, together with circular extractors.

Albucaſis has alſo given the draught of an inſtrument, which is both for opening and extracting the head; the point and wings are forced through the *Cranium*, and, when turned the contrary way, the two wings or hooks take hold of the inſide.

There are other later contrivances uſed and recommended by different gentlemen of the profeſſion, ſuch as *Mauriceau*'s tire-tête, *Simpſon*'s ſcalp-ring, and *Old*'s *Terebra occulta*, with the improvement made in it by Dr. *Burton* of *York*: and all theſe inſtruments may be uſed with ſucceſs if cautiouſly managed, ſo as not to injure the woman, except the *Speculum matricis*, which far from anſwering the ſuppoſed intention of it, namely, to extend the bones of the *Pelvis*, can ſerve no other purpoſe than that of bruiſing or inflaming the parts of the woman.

 The

The following method, if exactly followed according to the circumſtances of the caſe, ſeems, of all others hitherto invented, the eaſieſt, ſafeſt, and moſt certain; eſpecially when it requires great force to extract the head.

SECT. V.

The method of extracting with the CROTCHET.

WHEN the head preſents, and ſuch is the caſe, that the child can neither be delivered by turning, nor extracted with the forceps, and it is abſolutely neceſſary to deliver the woman to ſave her life, this operation muſt then be performed in the following manner.

The operator muſt be provided with a pair of curved crotchets, made according to the improvements upon thoſe propoſed by *Meſnard*, together with a pair of ſciſſars about nine inches long, with reſts near the middle of the blades, and the blunt hook.

NUMB.

NUMB. I.

Of the Woman's Posture.

THE patient ought to be laid on her back in the same position directed in the use of the forceps; the operator must be seated on a low chair, and the instruments concealed and disposed in the same manner, and for the same reason, mentioned in treating of the forceps. The parts of the woman have already, in all likelihood, been sufficiently dilated by his endeavours to turn or deliver with the forceps; or if no efforts of that kind have been used, because by the touch he had learned that no such endeavours would succeed, as in the case of a large hydrocephalus, when the bones of the *Cranium* are often separated at a great distance from each other; or upon perceiving that the *Pelvis* was extremely narrow. If upon these considerations he hath made no trials in which the parts were opened, let him gradually dilate the *Os externum* and *internum*, as formerly directed.

NUMB.

NUMB. II.

THE head is commonly kept down pretty firm by the ſtrong contraction of the *Uterus* round the child; but ſhould it yield to one ſide, let it be kept ſteady by the hand of an aſſiſtant, preſſing upon the belly of the woman: let him introduce his hand, and preſs two fingers againſt one of the ſutures of the *Cranium*; then take out his ſciſſars from the place in which they were depoſited, and guiding them by the hand and fingers till they reach the hairy ſcalp, then puſh them gradually into it until their progreſs is ſtopped by the reſts.

If the head ſlips aſide in ſuch a manner, as that they cannot be puſhed into the ſkull at the ſuture, they will make their way through the ſolid bones, if they are moved in a ſemicircular turn, like the motion of boring; and this method continued till you find the point firmly fixed, for if this is not obſerved, the points ſlide along the bones.

The ſciſſars ought to be ſo ſharp at the points, as to penetrate the integuments and bones when puſhed with a moderate force; but

but not ſo keen as to cut the operator's fingers, or the *Vagina*, in introducing them.

The ſciſſars being thus forced into the brain, as far as the reſts at the middle of the blades, let them be kept firm in that ſituation; and the hand that was in the *Vagina* being withdrawn, the operator muſt take hold of the handles with each hand and pull them aſunder, that the blades may dilate and make a large opening in the ſkull; then they muſt be ſhut, turned, and again pulled aſunder, ſo as to make the inciſion crucial; by which means, the opening will be enlarged, and ſufficient room made for the introduction of the fingers: let them be afterwards cloſed, and introduced even beyond the reſts, when they muſt again be opened, and turned half round from ſide to ſide, until the ſtructure of the brain is ſo effectually deſtroyed, that it can be evacuated with eaſe. This operation being performed, let the ſciſſars be ſhut and withdrawn; but if this inſtrument will not anſwer the laſt purpoſe, the buſineſs may be done by introducing the crotchet within the opening of the ſkull. The brain being thus de-

deſtroyed, and the inſtrument withdrawn, let him introduce his right hand into the *Vagina*, and two fingers into the opening which hath been made, that if any ſharp ſplinters of the bones remain, they may be broken off and taken out, leſt they ſhould injure the woman's *Vagina*, or the operator's own fingers.

NUMB. III.

IF the caſe be an hydrocephalus, let him fix his fingers on the inſide and his thumb on the outſide of the opening, and endeavour to pull along the ſkull in time of a pain; but if labour is weak, he muſt deſire the woman to aſſiſt his endeavours by forcing down: and thus the child is frequently delivered, becauſe the water being evacuated, the head collapſes of courſe.

NUMB. IV.

BUT when the *Pelvis* is narrow, the head requires much greater force to be brought along; unleſs the labour pains are ſtrong enough to preſs it down and diminiſh it, by ſqueezing out the *Cerebrum*: in

this

this caſe, let the operator withdraw his fingers from the opening, and ſlide them along the head, paſt the *Os uteri*, then, with his left hand taking one of the crotchets from the place of its concealment, introduce it along his right hand, with the point towards the child's head, and fix it above the chin, in the mouth, back part of the neck, or above the ears, or in any place where it will take firm hold; having fixed the inſtrument, let him withdraw his right hand, and with it take hold on the end or handle of the crotchet, then introduce his left to ſeize the bones at the opening of the ſkull (as above directed) that the head may be kept ſteady, and pull along with both hands.

If the head is ſtill detained by the uncommon narrowneſs of the *Pelvis*, let him introduce his left hand along the oppoſite ſide, in order to guide the other crotchet, which being alſo applied and locked or joined with its fellow, in the manner of the forceps, he muſt pull with ſufficient force, moving from ſide to ſide, and if the head does not preſent fair, turn the forehead into the hollow of the *Sacrum*, and extract as with the forceps,

ceps, humouring the ſhape of the head and *Pelvis*, during the operation, which ought to be performed ſlowly, with great judgment and caution; and from hence it appears abſolutely neceſſary to know how the head preſents, in order to judge how the crotchet muſt be fixed, and the head brought along to the beſt advantage.

Sometimes in theſe caſes, when I find that I cannot ſucceed, by pulling at the opening with my fingers; and if the woman has not had ſtrong pains, I introduce the ſmall end of the blunt hook into the opening, and placing my fingers againſt the point on the outſide of the ſkull, pull with greater and greater force; but as we can ſeldom take a firm hold in this manner, if it does not ſoon anſwer the purpoſe, I introduce my fingers as above, farther, and ſlide the point up along the outſide, above the under jaw; and have ſucceeded ſeveral times, with this inſtrument, except when the *Pelvis* was ſo narrow as to require a greater force; then we muſt uſe the others. No doubt, it is better firſt to try the blunt hook, becauſe the managing the point gives leſs

trouble,

trouble, and it can be eaſier introduced with the point to one ſide. When the inſtrument is far enough advanced, this point may be turned to the head, and as a very narrow *Pelvis* ſeldom occurs, the blunt hook will commonly ſucceed.

If, when the head is delivered in this manner, the body cannot be extracted, on account of its being much ſwelled, of a monſtrous ſize, or (which is moſt commonly the caſe) the narrowneſs of the *Pelvis*; let him deſiſt from pulling, leſt the head ſhould be ſeparated from the body, and introducing one hand ſo as to reach with his fingers to the ſhoulder blades or breaſt, conduct along it one of the crotchets, with the point towards the *Fœtus*, and fix it with a firm application; then withdrawing his hand, employ it in pulling the crotchet, while the other is exerted in the ſame manner, upon the head and neck of the child: if the inſtrument begins to loſe its hold, he muſt puſh it farther up, and fixing it again, repeat his efforts, applying it ſtill higher and higher, until the body is extracted.

Some writers direct us to introduce the crotchet within the ſkull, and preſſing one hand againſt the point on the outſide, pull along: but this is a trifling expedient, and if a good deal of force is uſed, the inſtrument tears through the thin bones, and hurts the operator's hand or the woman's *Vagina*, if not both. Whereas in the other method there is much more certainty; and a better purchaſe to force along the head, which collapſes, and is diminiſhed as the brain is diſcharged, and never comes down in a broad flattened form, according to the allegations of ſome people, whoſe ideas of theſe things are imperfect and confuſed: for if this were the caſe, the ſame would happen when the head is forced down from behind with labour pains, into a narrow *Pelvis*, becauſe the preſſure in both caſes, acts in the ſame direction; whereas we always find both in the one and the other, that the *Vertex* is protruded in a narrow point, and the whole head ſqueezed into a longiſh form.

Although many people have exclaimed againſt the crotchets as dangerous inſtruments, from ignorance, want of experience,

or

or a worſe principle, as formerly obſerved; yet I can aſſure the reader, that I never either tore or hurt the parts of a woman with that inſtrument. I have indeed ſeveral times hurt the inſide of my hand, by their giving way; till I had recourſe to the curve kind, which in many reſpects have the advantage of the ſtreight; and I am perſuaded, if managed as above directed, will never injure the patient.

Indeed young practitioners, 'till they are better informed by cuſtom and practice, may, after the head is opened, try to extract it with the ſmall or large forceps, and if it is not very large, or the *Pelvis* very narrow, they may deliver by ſqueezing and leſſening the head: but in my courſe of practice, I have been concerned in many caſes, where the *Pelvis* was ſo diſtorted and narrow, that even after opening the head largely, I have pulled at the bones, in time of ſtrong pains, but all to no purpoſe, although ſome of them actually came away. Nay, after fixing a crotchet firmly above, and near the chin or baſis of the ſcull, and uſing a good deal of force, I have not been able to move the head lower, till at laſt I have been obliged to introduce the other, and by intervals increaſe the force of pulling, to the utmoſt of my ſtrength; and before we had the curve crotchet, I have been ſo fatigued from the ſtreight kind ſlipping their ſmall hold ſo often, that I have ſcarcely been able to move my fingers or arms, for many hours after; and if this force had not been uſed, the mother muſt have been loſt as well as the child.

CHAP. IV.

Of PRÆTERNATURAL LABOURS.

SECT. I.

PRæternatural labour, according to the diviſion mentioned, chap. I. ſect. 5. happens, when inſtead of the head, ſome other part of the body preſents to the *Os uteri*. It has been thought by ſome, that all labours in which the forceps and crotchet are uſed, ought to be ranked in this claſs; becauſe the head is certainly delivered by præter-

præternatural means; and that when the feet or breech preſent, and the woman is delivered without any other aſſiſtance than that of labour pains, the caſe ought to be accounted natural. However, this diviſion would embarraſs and confuſe young beginners, more than the other which I have choſen to follow, namely that of reckoning by the manner in which the child is delivered, and calling all thoſe births præternatural, in which the body is delivered before the head. Præternatural labours are more or leſs difficult according to the preſentation of the child, and the contraction of the *Uterus* round its body. The nearer the head and ſhoulders are to the *Os internum*, or lower part of the *Uterus*, the more difficult is the caſe; whereas when the head is towards the *Fundus*, and the feet or breech near the *Os internum*, it is more eaſy to turn and deliver.

To begin with the eaſieſt of theſe firſt, it may be proper to divide them into three claſſes. Firſt, how to manage when the feet, breech, or lower parts preſent. Secondly, how to behave in violent floodings; and when the child presents wrong before the membranes are broke, how to save the waters in the *Uterus*, that the *Fœtus* may be the more easily turned; and what method to follow even after the membranes are broke, when all the waters are not evacuated. Thirdly, how to deliver when the *Uterus* is strongly contracted, the child presenting either with the fore or back parts, and lying in a circular form; or with the shoulders, breast, neck, face, ear, or *Vertix*, and lying in a longish form, with the feet and breech towards the *Fundus* of the womb, which is contracted like a long sheath, close to the body of the *Fœtus*; and when the foreparts of the child lie towards the side, *Fundus*, fore or back part of the *Uterus*. *Daventer*, who practised at *Dort* in *Holland*, alledges that præternatural as well as laborious cases proceed from the wrong position of the *Os* and *Fundus uteri*; that if the *Fundus* hangs forwards over the *Pubis*, the *Os uteri* is turned backwards towards the *Sacrum*, and that in whatsoever direction the *Fundus* inclines, the *Os uteri* will be always turned to the opposite side. This opinion he grounded upon the ſuppoſition, that the *Placenta* always adheres to the *Fundus*: but experience ſhews, that it adheres to different parts of the womb, ſometimes even to the inſide of the *Os uteri*. For the moſt part, indeed, the *Os internum* is turned backwards towards the *Coccyx*, being in a ſtreight line with the *Fundus* up to the middle ſpace betwixt the navel and *Scrobiculum cordis*.

Daventer was alſo of opinion, that if, upon touching, the mouth of the womb was not felt in the middle, the woman ought to be aſſiſted by opening the parts; and if this did not ſucceed, by turning and delivering by the feet without delay. We ſometimes, indeed, meet with pendulous bellies, in which the *Os uteri* is farther back than uſual; but, even in theſe caſes, when the head is not very large, nor the *Pelvis* narrow, and the woman is vigorous and the labour-pains ſtrong, the woman with a little patience, is, for the moſt part, ſafely delivered without any other than common aſſiſtance: or ſhould the caſe prove tedious, ſhe may be aſſiſted in time of a pain by introducing one or two fingers into the *Os uteri*, and gradually bringing it more forwards. When the belly is very pendulous, change of poſition from time to time is of ſervice, eſpecially lying upon her back with the ſhoulders low and the breech raiſed.

In women that are diſtorted, when one *Ilium* is much lower than the other, the *Fundus uteri* will be turned to the low ſide; but there the chief difficulty will proceed from the narrowneſs of the *Pelvis*.

SECT. II.

The firſt Claſs of PRÆTERNATURAL LABOURS. *When the Feet, Breech, or lower parts of the* Fœtus *preſent, and the Head, Shoulders, and upper parts are towards the* Fundus.

THESE, for the moſt part, are accounted the eaſieſt, even although the *Uterus* ſhould be ſtrongly contracted round the body of the child, and all the waters diſcharged.

If the knees or feet of the child preſent to the *Os internum*, which is not yet ſufficiently dilated to allow them and the body to come farther down; or if the woman is weak,

wore

wore out with long labour, or endangered by a flooding, let the operator introduce his hand into the *Vagina*, puſh up and ſtretch the *Os uteri*, and bring along the feet; which being extracted, let him wrap a linnen cloth round them, and pull until the breech appears on the outſide of the *Os externum*: if the face or fore part of the *Fœtus* is already towards the back of the *Uterus*, let him perſiſt in pulling in the ſame direction; but if they are towards the *Pubis*, or one ſide, they muſt be turned to the back-part of the *Uterus*, and as the head does not move round equal with the body, he muſt make allowance for the difference in turning, by bringing the laſt one quarter farther than the place at which the head is to be placed; ſo that the face or forehead which was towards one of the groins, will be forced to the ſide of the *Sacrum*, where it joins with the *Iſchium*. This quarter turn of the body muſt be again undone, without affecting the poſition of the head; a cloth may be wrapped round the breech, for the convenience of holding it more firmly; then placing a thumb along each ſide of the ſpine, and with his fingers graſping the belly, let him pull along the body from ſide to ſide, with more or leſs force, according to the reſiſtance: when the child is delivered as far as the ſhoulders, let him ſlide his hand flattened (ſuppoſe the right, if lying on her back) between its breaſt and the *Perineum*, *Coccyx*, and *Sacrum* of the woman, and introduce the fore or middle finger (or both, if neceſſary) into the mouth of the *Fœtus*; by which means the chin will be pulled to the breaſt, and the forehead into the hollow of the *Sacrum*. And this expedient will alſo raiſe upwards the hindhead, which reſts at the *Pubis*.

When the forehead is come ſo low as to protrude the *Perineum*, if the woman lies on her back, let the operator ſtand up, and pull the body and head of the child upwards, bringing the forehead with an half-round turn from the under part of the *Os externum*, which will thus be defended from laceration. The application of the fingers in the child's mouth will contribute to bring the head out in this manner, prevent the *Os externum* from hitching on the chin, help along the head, and guard the neck from being over-ſtrained;

a

a misfortune which would infallibly happen, if the forehead ſhould be detained at the upper-part of the *Sacrum:* nor is there any great force required to obviate this inconvenience, or the leaſt danger of hurting the child's mouth, if not large; for if the head cannot be brought along with moderate force, and the operator is afraid of injuring or overſtraining the lower jaw, let him puſh his fingers farther up, and preſs on each ſide of the noſe, or on the inferior edges of the ſockets of the eyes. If the legs are come out, and the breech pulled into the *Vagina*, there is no occaſion for puſhing up to open, but only to pull along and manage as above directed; ſtill remembering to raiſe the forehead ſlowly from the *Perineum*, which may be preſſed back with the fingers of his other hand.

In the caſe of a narrow *Pelvis*, or large head, which cannot be brought along without the riſk of over-ſtraining the neck, let him ſlide up his fingers and hand into the *Vagina*, and bring down one of the child's arms, at the ſame time pulling the body to the contrary ſide, by which means the ſhoulder will

will be brought lower down: let him run his fingers along the arm until they reach the elbow, which muſt be pulled downwards with an half-round turn to the other ſide, below the breaſt. This muſt not be done with a jirk, but ſlowly and cautiouſly, in order to prevent the diſlocation, bending, or breaking of the child's arm.

Let him again guide his fingers into the child's mouth, and try if the head will come along: if this will not ſucceed, let the body be pulled to the other ſide, ſo as to bring down the other ſhoulder; then ſlide up his left hand, and extracting the other arm, endeavour to deliver the head. If one finger of his right hand be fixed in the child's mouth, let the body reſt on that arm; let him place the left hand above the ſhoulders, and put a finger on each ſide of the neck: if the forehead is towards one ſide at the upper-part of the *Pelvis*, let him pull it lower down, and gradually turn it into the hollow of the *Sacrum*; then ſtand up, and in pulling raiſe the body, ſo as to bring out the head in an half-round turn, as above directed.

Da-

Daventer, and others, from a miſtaken notion, that the chief reſiſtance is at the *Coccyx* or lower part of the *Pelvis*, have directed us to preſs the ſhoulders of the child downwards, ſo as to bring the hindhead firſt from below the *Pubis*; not conſidering that the reſiſtance is occaſioned by the thickeſt part of the head being detained at the upper-part of the *Pelvis*, where the loweſt *Vertebra* of the loins, and the upper-part of the *Sacrum* jet inwards; and that until the forehead hath paſſed into the hollow of the *Sacrum*, this method cannot ſucceed: the buſineſs, therefore, is to pull upwards at the back-part of the neck, which reſts againſt the under-part of the *Pubis*, and by this exertion the forehead, which is high up, will be brought down with a circular turn; after which the head ſeldom ſtops, and the ſame circular motion is ſtill the moſt proper, though now we can bring out the head the other way, but not before. Sometimes, indeed, I have found *Daventer*'s method ſucceed better than the other, when the head is low down, and the chief reſiſtance is in the lower parts; but this is very ſeldom the caſe: how-

however, when the forehead is hindered from coming down into the lower part of the *Sacrum* by an uncommon ſhape of the head or *Pelvis*, and we cannot extract it by bringing it out with an half-round turn at the *Pubis*, we muſt try to make this turn in the contrary direction; and inſtead of introducing our fingers into the child's mouth, let the breaſt of it reſt on the palm of your left hand, (the woman being on her back) and placing the right on its ſhoulders, with the fingers on each ſide of the neck, preſs it downwards to the *Perineum*. In conſequence of this preſſure, the face and chin being within the *Perineum*, will move more upwards, and the head come out with an half-round turn from below the *Os pubis*: for the center of motion is now where the fore-part of the neck preſſes at the *Perineum*; whereas, in the other method, the back-part of the neck is againſt the lower part of the *Pubis*, on which the head turns.

If the forehead is not turned to one ſide, but ſticks at the upper-part of the *Sacrum*, eſpecially when the *Pelvis* is narrow; let him endeavour with his finger in the mouth

to

to turn it to one ſide of the jetting in of the *Sacrum*, becauſe the *Pelvis* is wider at the ſides of the brim, and bring it along as before.

If one of the child's arms, inſtead of being placed along the ſides of the head, are turned in between the face and *Sacrum*, or between the hindhead and *Pubis*, the ſame difficulty of extracting occurs, as in a large head or narrow *Pelvis*; and this poſition frequently enſues when the fore-parts of the child's body are turned from the *Pubis* down to the *Sacrum*: If they are turned to the left ſide of the woman, the left hand and arm are commonly brought in before the face, and *vice verſa*; but in theſe caſes, the elbow is, for the moſt part, eaſily come at, becauſe it is low down in the *Vagina*, and then there is a neceſſity for bringing down one or both arms before the head can be delivered: from whence we may conclude, that thoſe authors are ſometimes in the wrong, who expreſly forbid us to pull down the arms. Indeed if the *Pelvis* is not narrow, nor the head very large, and the arms lie along the ſides of the head, there is ſeldom occaſion to pull them down; becauſe the *Pelvis* is wideſt at the ſides, and the membranes and ligaments that fill up the ſpace betwixt the *Sacrum* and *Iſchia*, yield to the preſſure, and make room for the paſſage of the head: but when they are ſqueezed between the head and *Sacrum*, *Iſchia*, or *Pubis*, and the head ſticks in the *Pelvis*, they certainly ought to be brought down; or even when the head comes along with difficulty. Neither is the alledged contraction of the *Os internum* round the neck of the child, ſo frequent as hath been imagined; becauſe, for the moſt part, the contraction embraces the head and not the neck: but ſhould the neck alone ſuffer, that inconvenience may be removed by introducing the hand into the *Vagina*, and a finger or two into the child's mouth: by which means alſo a ſufficient dilatation will be preſerved in the *Os externum*, which frequently contracts on the neck as ſoon as the arms are brought out.

The diſtance from the face or forehead to the *Vertix* being greater than that from the forehead to the back-part of the hindhead or neck, when the hindhead reſts at the *Pubis*, and

and the forehead at the upper part of the *Sacrum*, the head can ſeldom be brought down until the operator, by introducing a finger into the mouth, moves the ſame to the ſide, brings the chin to the breaſt, and the forehead into the hollow of the *Sacrum*; by which means the hindhead is raiſed and allowed to come along with greater eaſe: and in pulling, half the force only is applied to the neck, the other half being exerted upon the head by the finger which is fixed in the mouth; ſo that the forehead is more eaſily brought out by pulling upwards, with the half-round turn from the *Perineum*. When the operator, with his fingers in the child's mouth, cannot pull down the forehead into the hollow of the *Sacrum*, let him puſh the fore finger of his left hand betwixt the neck and *Pubis*, in order to raiſe the hindhead upwards; which being done, the forehead will come down with leſs difficulty, eſpecially if he puſhes up and pulls down at the ſame time, or alternately.

If it be diſcovered by the touch, that the breech preſents, that the membranes are not yet broke, the woman in no danger, the *Os* in-

internum not yet ſufficiently dilated, and the labour-pains ſtrong; the midwife ought to wait until the membranes, with the waters, are puſhed farther down, as in the natural labour: for, as they come down through the *Os uteri* into the *Vagina*, they ſtretch open the parts contained in the *Pelvis*, and the bulk within the *Uterus* being diminiſhed, it contracts and comes in contact with the body of the child; ſo that the breech is puſhed along by the mechanical force of the abdominal muſcles operating upon the womb.

The ſame conſequence will follow even although the membranes are broke; for the waters lubricate the parts as they flow off, and the breech, if not too large, or the *Pelvis* narrow, is puſhed down: In this caſe, when the *Nates* preſent equal and fair to the *Os uteri*, (as was formerly obſerved when treating of the poſition of the child, book III. chap. 1. ſect. 1. it was moſt probable, that one ſide of the *Fœtus* was towards the fore-part, and the other to the back-part of the *Uterus*;) ſo it is alſo reaſonable to conclude, that when the breech preſents, it lies in the ſame manner, but that the fore-parts of the child

child are rather turned backwards to one ſide of the *Vertebra* of the loins: in this poſition one hip will preſent, and the other reſt on the *Os pubis*; but when forced along with pains, the laſt will be gradually moved more and more to the groin of that ſide, and from thence ſlip down at the ſide of the baſin: the lower at the ſame time will be forced to the other, and the hollow betwixt the thighs will reſt upon the jetting-in of the *Os ſacrum*, and come down in that manner; the thighs on each ſide, and the back and round part of the breech paſſing in below the arch of the *Os pubis*, which is the beſt poſition: but if the back of the child is tilted backwards, then it will be forced down in the contrary direction, and come along with more difficulty, *viz.* the thighs to the *Pubis*, and back to the *Sacrum*: when it is come down to the middle or lower part of the *Pelvis*, let the operator introduce the forefinger of each hand along the outſide, to the groins, and taking hold, pull gently along, during a ſtrong pain.

If the *Os externum* is ſo contracted, that he cannot take ſufficient hold, let it be opened ſlowly, ſo as to allow his hands to be puſhed up with eaſe; when he has inſinuated a finger or two in each groin, let him place his thumbs on the thighs, if they are towards the *Pubis*, ſo as to obtain a firm hold; then pull along from ſide to ſide, and if the back of the child is to the *Pubis*, continue to aſſiſt in this manner, until the body and head are delivered: the legs being commonly ſtretched up along the belly and breaſt, when the child is extracted as far as the ſhoulders, they come out of themſelves, or are eaſily brought down; but if the belly of the child is turned to one ſide, or to the *Pubis*, in that caſe, when the breech is delivered, he ought to turn the belly down to the *Sacrum*, and the back to the *Pubis*; and that the face may be alſo turned to the back of the mother, let him remember the quarter extraordinary, which muſt be again reverſed, and then he may pull along, and deliver.

If the body cannot be turned, until the thighs and legs are brought down, either on account of the bulk, or becauſe the hold on the breech is not ſufficient, let him continue to pull along, until the hams appear on the outſide of the *Os externum*; then ſeize one of the knees with his finger and thumb, and extract that leg; and let the other be brought down in the ſame manner. If he attempts to pull out the legs, before the hams arrive at this place, the thighs are always in danger of being bent or broke. When the legs are delivered, let him wrap a cloath round the breech of the child, and as the body was pulled down almoſt as far as the breaſt, before the legs could be brought out, it muſt be puſhed up again to the navel, or above it; becauſe, without this precaution, the ſhoulders would be ſo much engaged in the *Pelvis*, that it would be impracticable to make the motions formerly directed, ſo as to turn the face to the back of the mother; whereas, when the body is puſhed up, thoſe turns can be effected with greater eaſe, becauſe the belly being in the *Pelvis*, it yields eaſier to the form of the baſin. When the face is turned properly down, let him proceed to deliver, as above directed.

If the breech is detained above the *Pelvis*, either by its uncommon magnitude, or the narrowneſs of the baſin; or if one of the *Nates* is puſhed in, while the other reſts above the *Pubis*, *Sacrum*, or to either ſide; if the woman is low and weak, the pains lingering and inſufficient to force the child along; or if ſhe is in danger from a violent flooding: in any of theſe caſes, let him (during every pain) gradually open, firſt the *Os externum*, and then the *Os internum*, with his fingers and hand. Having thus gained admiſſion, let him puſh up the breech to the fore or back part, or to one ſide of the *Uterus*, that his hand and arm may have room to ſlide along the foreparts or belly of the child, ſo as to feel the thighs, that will direct him to the legs, which muſt be brought down with his fingers, while at the ſame time, he puſhes up the hams with his thumb, that in caſe the legs lie ſtreight up, they may be extracted with more eaſe by the flection of the knee, and run the leſs riſk of being bent, broke, or overſtrained: for if they are folded downward, they are the more eaſily brought out.

If the breech be ſtrongly preſſed into the upper part of the *Pelvis*, let him alſo puſh it upwards and to one ſide, that his hand and arm may have free paſſage; for, the higher

higher the breech is raiſed out of his way, he will be at more freedom to extract the legs.

If both legs cannot be eaſily brought down, he may ſafely deliver with one, of which taking hold with a linnen cloth wrapped round it, let him ſlide up his other hand into the *Vagina*, and a finger or two into the outſide of the groin which is bent: by theſe means, the hip will come down the eaſier, and the leg which is already extracted will not be overſtrained by ſuſtaining the whole force of pulling the body along.

If the legs lie towards the left ſide of the woman, who is laid on her back, the right hand muſt be introduced into the *Uterus*: if they lie to her right ſide, the left hand will better anſwer the purpoſe; and if they are towards her back or belly, either hand may be indifferently uſed.

In all caſes where the breech preſents, the ſafeſt practice is always to puſh up and bring down the legs, provided the *Os uteri* is ſufficiently dilated, and the waters not wholly diſcharged. If the waters are evacuated, the *Uterus* ſtrongly contracted around the child, the breech low, ſo as that it cannot be returned, or ſo ſmall as to come eaſily along, we ought then to deliver it accordingly; but if ſo large as neither to be puſhed up or brought along with the aſſiſtance of the fingers, let the operator introduce the curved handle of the blunt crotchet into one of the groins, his fingers into the other, and pull very cautiouſly, in order to prevent a fracture or diſlocation of the thigh bone, which might otherwiſe happen from the uſe of this inſtrument, the blunt point of which muſt be ſufficiently paſt the groin. A fillet may alſo be uſed for the ſame purpoſe.

I have in the foregoing caſes of this ſection, ſuppoſed the woman laid on her back, her legs ſupported, and breech to the bedſide; this being generally the beſt poſition for delivering the body and head: indeed, when the child is ſmall, ſhe may lie on her ſide, and the ſame methods uſed in delivering, provided the operator ſtill remembers, that in this poſition, the *Ilium* and *Iſchium* of one ſide is down, and the others up. Beſides, when the breech is puſhed up, in order

der

der to bring down the legs, if they lie forwards towards the forepart of the *Uterus*, and the belly is pendulous, he can reach them with the greateſt eaſe, when ſhe lies on one ſide: but when the legs are delivered, if the child is large or the *Pelvis* narrow, ſhe ought to be turned upon her back, becauſe the body and head can be better and ſafer delivered, by pulling up and down and in that poſture ſhe is alſo kept more firm, and her thighs leſs in the operator's way, than when ſhe lies upon her ſide.

SECT. III.

The ſecond claſs of PRÆTERNATURAL LABOURS.

WHEN the membranes are broke, but the face, ſhoulder or ſome other part of the child being puſhed into the *Pelvis*, locks up the *Os internum* ſo as that a ſmall quantity of the waters hath been diſcharged, the *Uterus* is kept from contracting ſtrongly round the child, which is therefore more eaſily turned than it poſſibly can be when they are all gone:

When, before the membranes are broke the child is felt through them, presenting wrong, and at the same time the pains push them down so as to dilate the *Os internum*, more or less:

When the woman, at any time in the four last months, is seized with a violent flooding that cannot be restrained, and unless speedily delivered must lose her life; if labour-pains cannot be brought on by stretching the parts, delivery must be forced; but if she is in labour, and the membranes have been pushed down with the waters, they may be broke; by which means the flooding is frequently diminished and the child delivered by the labour-pains.

In these three different cases, if we can prevent the strong contraction of the *Uterus*, by keeping up the waters, we can also for the most part turn the child with great ease, even in the very worst positions.

Numb. I.

In the first case, let the operator slowly introduce his hand into the *Vagina*, and his fingers between that part of the child which is pushed down, and the *Os internum*: if in so doing he perceives some of the waters coming along, he must run up his hand as quick as possible into the *Uterus*, betwixt the inside of the membranes and the child's body; the lower part of his arm will then fill up the *Os externum* like a plug, so that no more of the waters can pass; let him turn the child with its head and shoulders up to the *Fundus*, the breech down to the lower part of the *Uterus*, and the foreparts towards the mother's back; let the hand be pushed no farther up than the middle of the child's body, because, if it is advanced as high as the *Fundus*, it must be withdrawn lower, before the child can be turned; and by these means the waters will be discharged, and the *Uterus* of consequence contract so as to render the turning more difficult.

NUMB. II.

IN the second case, when the membranes are not broke, and we are certain that the child does not present fair, if the *Os internum* is not sufficiently dilated, and the woman in no danger, we may let the labour

go

go on, until the parts are more ſtretched; lubricating and extending the *Os externum*, by degrees, during every pain. Then introducing one hand into the *Vagina*, we inſinuate it in a flattened form, within the *Os internum*, and puſh up between the membranes and the *Uterus*, as far as the middle of the womb: having thus obtained admiſſion, we break the membranes by graſping and ſqueezing them with our fingers, ſlide our hand within them, without moving the arm lower down, then turn and deliver as formerly directed.

NUMB. III.

IF the woman (in the third caſe) is attacked with a violent flooding, occaſioned by a ſeparation of all or any part of the *Placenta* from the *Uterus*, during the laſt four months of pregnancy, and every method has in vain been tried to leſſen and reſtrain the diſcharge, according to the directions in book II. chap. 3. ſect. 3. the operator ought to pronounce the caſe dangerous, and prudently declare to the relations of the patient, that unleſs ſhe is ſpeedily delivered, both ſhe

and

and the child muſt periſh, obſerving, at the ſame time, that by immediate delivery they may both be ſaved; let him alſo deſire the aſſiſtance and advice of ſome perſon eminent in the profeſſion, for the ſatisfaction of her friends and the ſupport of his own reputation. When there are no labour pains, and the mouth of the womb is not dilated, it is ſometimes very difficult to deliver, more eſpecially if the *Os internum* is not a little lax, but feels rigid.

If the *Os uteri* is ſo much contracted, that the finger cannot be introduced, ſome authors have recommended a dilator, by which it may be gradually opened ſo as to admit a finger or two. Doubtleſs, ſome caſes may happen, in which this may be neceſſary: though in all thoſe to which I have been called, when there was a neceſſity for forcing delivery, the mouth of the womb was open enough to receive the tip of my finger, ſo that by gradual efforts I could effect a ſufficient dilatation; and it is certainly a ſafer method to dilate with the fingers and hand, than with an inſtrument. If in ſtretching the *Os internum*, labour-pains

pains are brought on, let the operator ſlowly proceed and encourage them: when the mouth of the womb is opened, if the head preſents and the pains are ſtrong, by breaking the membranes the flooding will be diminiſhed; but if ſhe floods to ſuch a degree as to be in danger of her life, and the dilatation does not bring on labour, at leaſt not enough for the occaſion, ſhe muſt be immediately delivered in the following manner: but in the firſt place let her friends be apprized of the danger, and the operator beware of promiſing to ſave either mother or child; for I have known the woman die in a few minutes after delivery, although to all appearance ſhe ſeemed able to undergo the operation, and the child loſt from the head's ſticking in the *Pelvis*. Others again, who were apparently much more weak and exhauſted, have recovered, and the child hath been ſaved.

The operator having performed his duty in making the friends acquainted with the ſituation of the caſe, muſt gently open the *Os externum*, by introducing his fingers gradually, turning them half round and puſhing upwards; then forming them, with the thumb, into the figure of a wedge or cone, continue to dilate ſlowly and by intervals, until his hand is admitted into the *Vagina*: having thus far gained his point, let him inſinuate, in the ſame ſlow cautious manner, firſt one, then two fingers, into the *Os internum*, which may be dilated ſo as to admit the other two and the thumb in the ſame conical form, which will gradually make way for ſliding the hand along between the outſide of the membranes and inſide of the *Uterus*; then he muſt manage as directed in the ſecond caſe. If upon ſliding up his hand upon the outſide of the membranes, he feels the *Placenta* adhering to that ſide of the womb, he muſt either withdraw that hand and introduce the other on the oppoſite ſide, or break through the membranes at the lower edge of the *Placenta*.

The greateſt danger in this caſe frequently proceeds from the ſudden emptying of the *Uterus* and belly; for when labour comes on of itſelf, or is brought on in a regular manner, and the membranes are broke, the flooding is gradually diminiſhed, and firſt the

 child,

child, then the *Placenta*, is delivered by the pains: ſo that the preſſure or reſiſtance is not all at once removed from the belly and *Uterus* of the woman, which have time to contract by degrees; conſequently thoſe fainting fits and convulſions are prevented which often proceed from a ſudden removal of that compreſſion, under which the circulation was performed.

In order to anticipate theſe fatal ſymptoms, I have (ſometimes ſucceſsfully) ordered an aſſiſtant to preſs upon the woman's belly while the *Uterus* was emptying; or, after having broke the membranes, turned up the head to the *Fundus*, and brought down the legs and breech, I withdraw my arm a little, to let the waters come off, though I keep my hand in the *Uterus* for a few minutes, and do not extract the legs until I feel the womb cloſe contracted to the child; nay, if the flooding is ſtopped or even diminiſhed, I let the child remain in the *Uterus* perhaps ten or fifteen minutes longer, then deliver; and if the hæmorrhage is ſtayed, leave the *Placenta* to be expelled by nature. In all theſe ſtages, however, when

when the flooding is violent, we muſt deliver without loſs of time, remembering ſtill the preſſure upon the abdomen; for the woman is frequently ſo very weak, that although labour could be brought on, ſhe would not have ſtrength ſufficient to undergo it.

The younger the woman is with child, the greater is the difficulty in opening the *Os internum*; and more ſo in the firſt child, eſpecially if ſhe is paſt the age of thirty-five.

We ſhould never refuſe to deliver in theſe dangerous caſes, even although the patient ſeems expiring: for immediately after delivery, the *Uterus* contracts, the mouths of the veſſels are ſhut up; ſo that the flooding ceaſes, and ſhe may recover, if ſhe lives five or ſix hours after the operation, and can be ſupported by frequent draughts of broth, gelly, caudle, weak cordial, and anodyne medicines, which maintain the circulation and gradually fill the empty veſſels.

If in time of flooding, ſhe is ſeized with labour-pains, or if by every now and then ſtretching with your fingers the *Os internum*, you bring on labour, by which either the membranes or head of the child is puſhed

down,

down, and opens the *Os internum*, the membranes ought to be broke; ſo that ſome of the waters being diſcharged, the *Uterus* may contract and ſqueeze down the *Fœtus*. This may be done ſooner in thoſe women who have had children formerly, than in ſuch as have never been in labour before. If, notwithſtanding this expedient, the flooding ſtill continues, and the child is not like to be ſoon delivered, it muſt be turned immediately; or if the head is in the *Pelvis* delivered with the forceps: but if neither of theſe two methods will ſucceed, on account of the narrowneſs of the *Pelvis*, or the bigneſs of the head, this laſt muſt be opened, and delivered with the crotchet. In all theſe caſes, let the parts be dilated ſlowly and by intervals, in order to prevent laceration.

SECT. IV.

The third Claſs of PRÆTERNATURAL LABOURS.

WE have already obſerved, that the principal difficulties in turning children and bringing them by the feet, proceeded from the

the contraction of the *Uterus* and bad position of the *Fœtus*. If the child lies in a round form, whether the fore-parts are towards the *Os internum* or *Fundus uteri*, we can for the most part move it with the hand, so as to turn the head and shoulders to the upper part, and the breech and legs downwards; but if the child lies lengthways, the womb being contracted around it, like a long sheath, the task is more difficult; especially if the head and shoulders of the child are down at the lowest part of the *Uterus*, with the breech and feet turned up to the *Fundus*.

Before I proceed to the method of delivery in the following cases, it will not be improper to premise, that the woman ought to be laid on her back, her breech upon the side or foot of the bed, a bolster or pillows being laid between the feather-bed or matress, in order to raise it so as that the breech may be higher than the shoulders; while an assistant sits on each side to support her legs and thighs, as directed in chap. II. sect. 1. and chap. III. sect. 3. and one or two more assistants ought to sit behind, or on each side of her ſhoulders, to keep her firm in that poſition. The operator ought to avoid all formality in point of dreſs, and never walk about the room with ſleeves and apron; for although ſuch apparatus may be neceſſary in hoſpitals, in private practice it conveys a frightful idea to the patient and female ſpectators: the more genteel and commodious dreſs is, a looſe waſhing night-gown, which he may always have in readineſs to put on when he is going to deliver; his waiſtcoat ought to be without ſleeves, ſo that his arms may have more freedom to ſlide up and down under cover of the wrapper; and the ſleeves of his ſhirt may be rolled up and pinned to the breaſts of his waiſtcoat. In natural labours, the ſheet that hangs over the bed-ſide is ſufficient to keep him clean and dry, by being laid upon his lap; but, in thoſe caſes where he is obliged to alter his poſition, a ſheet ought to be tucked round him, or an apron put on, but not before he is about to begin his work. If the patient is laid on a low bed, and he intends to introduce his right hand, his beſt and firmeſt poſition is to kneel with his left knee on a cuſhion,

 keep-

keeping up the right to ſupport his arm; if the left hand is introduced, the reverſe of this diſpoſition muſt take place: if the bed or couch is high, he ought to ſtand, but ſtill remember to ſupport the elbow on the knee. Theſe directions, howſoever trivial they may ſeem to old practitioners, may be ſerviceable to young beginners.

The hand of the accoucheur or operator being introduced into the *Uterus*, if he finds the breech below the head and ſhoulders, let him ſearch for the legs and bring them down; but if the breech be higher than the upper parts of the child, or equal with them, he muſt try to turn the head and ſhoulders to the *Fundus*, and the breech downwards, by puſhing up the firſt, and pulling down the laſt; then proceed with delivery as before directed. This is commonly executed with eaſe, provided ſome part of the waters ſtill remain in the *Uterus*; but if the woman has been long in labour, and the waters diſcharged, the contraction of the womb is ſo ſtrong, that the child cannot be turned without the exertion of great force frequently repeated. In this caſe, the eaſieſt method both for the patient and operator, is to puſh up the hand gradually on that ſide to which the legs and thighs are turned, and even after he has reached them, if they are not very high up, let him advance his hand as far as the *Fundus uteri*; he will thus remove the greateſt obſtacle, by enlarging the cavity of the womb, ſo as more eaſily to feel and bring down the legs; then he may puſh up and pull down, as we have preſcribed above: but if the head and ſhoulders ſtill continue to hinder the breech and body from coming along, and the feet cannot be brought ſo low as the outſide of the *Os externum*, while they are yet in the *Vagina* he may apply a nooſe upon one or both; for unleſs the child is ſo ſmall that he can turn it round by graſping the body when the head and ſhoulders are puſhed up, and he endeavours to bring down the other parts, they will again return to the ſame place, and retard delivery: whereas if he gains a firm hold of the feet, either without the *Os externum*, or in the *Vagina*, by means of the nooſe fixed upon the ancles, he can with the other hand puſh up the head and ſhoulder, and be able in that man-

ner

ner to bring down the breech. He muſt continue this method of puſhing up and pulling down, until the head and ſhoulder are raiſed to the *Fundus uteri*; for ſhould he leave off too ſoon, and withdraw his hand, although the child is extracted as far as the breech, the head is ſometimes ſo preſſed down and engaged with the body in the paſſage, that it cannot be brought farther down without being tore along with the crotchet: for the breech and part of the body may block up the paſſage in ſuch a manner, as that the hand cannot be introduced to raiſe the head.

In all caſes where the accoucheur foreſees that great force will be requiſite, he ought to ſave his ſtrength as much as poſſible, beginning ſlowly, and reſting his hand between whiles, during the operation of puſhing up and turning the child in the *Uterus*: for, if he begins to work in an hurry, and exerts his utmoſt ſtrength at firſt, his hands will be ſo cramped and enervated, that he will be obliged to deſiſt, and give them ſome reſpite; ſo that it may be a long time before he recovers the uſe of them, and even then they

 will

will be ſo much weakened as to be ſcarce able to effect delivery, which is thus impeded and delayed.

Thoſe caſes are commonly the eaſieſt in which the fore-parts preſent, and the child lies in a round or oval form, acroſs the *Uterus*, or diagonally, when the head or breech are above and over the *Pubis*, with the legs, arms, and navel-ſtring, or one or all of them, at the upper or lower part of the *Vagina*, or on the outſide of the *Os externum*. Thoſe are more difficult in which, though the child lies in the ſame round or contracted form, the back, ſhoulders, belly, or breaſt, are over the *Os internum*; becauſe, if we cannot move the child round, ſo as to place the head to the *Fundus*, the legs are brought down with much more difficulty than in the other caſe: but if the ſhoulder, breaſt, neck, ear, face, or crown of the head preſents, and the legs and breech are up to the *Fundus uteri*, the caſe is ſtill more difficult; becauſe in the other two, the *Uterus* is contracted in a round form, ſo that the wrong poſition of the child is more eaſily altered than in this, when the womb is contracted

tracted in a long ſhape, and ſometimes requires vaſt force to ſtretch it, ſo as that the head may be raiſed to the *Fundus*, and the legs and breech brought down.

The crown of the head is the worſt part that can preſent, becauſe in that caſe the feet and breech are higher, and the *Uterus* of a longer form, than in any other. The preſentation of the face is, next to this, attended with the greateſt difficulty: but when the neck, ſhoulder, back, or breaſt preſent, the head is turned upwards, and keeps the lower part of the womb diſtended; ſo that, upon ſtretching the upper part, the child's head is more eaſily raiſed to the *Fundus*.

Numb. I.

When the fore-parts of the child preſent, if the feet, hands, and navel-ſtring are not detained above the *Os uteri*, ſome or all of them deſcend into the *Vagina*, or appear on the outſide of the *Os externum*. If one or more of them come down, and the child at the ſame time lies in a round form acroſs the *Uterus*, let the accoucheur introduce his hand between them and the *Sacrum*, as directed

 in

in ſect. 3. When it is paſt the *Os internum*, let it reſt a little, while he feels with his fingers the poſition of the *Fœtus*: if the head and ſhoulders lie higher than the breech, he muſt take hold of the legs and bring them down withoutſide the *Os externum*: if the breech is detained above the brim of the *Pelvis*, let him ſlide up the flat of his hand along the buttocks, and pull down the legs with the other hand; by which method the breech is diſengaged and forced into the middle of the *Pelvis*.

In moſt of thoſe caſes where the child is preſt in an oval form, if neither the head or breech preſent, the head is to one ſide of the *Uterus*, and the breech to the other; becauſe, as was formerly obſerved, it is wider from ſide to ſide, than from the back to the fore part, and if either the head or breech is over the *Os pubis*, the other is turned off to the ſide: in moving the head or ſhoulders to the *Fundus*, they are raiſed with greater eaſe along the ſides, than at the back or fore parts, for the ſame reaſons.

If the head and ſhoulders lie lower down, ſo as to hinder the breech from coming

along,

along, and the legs from being extracted, let him puſh up the head and ſhoulders to the *Fundus*, and pull out the legs; then try as above directed to bring in the breech, and if it ſtill ſticks above, becauſe the head and ſhoulders are again forced down by the contraction of the *Uterus*, he muſt with one hand take hold of the legs that are now without the *Os externum*, and ſliding the other into the *Uterus*, puſh the head and ſhoulders again up to the *Fundus*, while, at the ſame time, he pulls the legs and breech along with the feet. If the legs cannot be brought farther down than the *Vagina*, becauſe the breech is high up, let him ſlip a nooſe over the feet round the ancles, as before obſerved; by which he may pull down the lower parts with one hand, while the other is employed in puſhing up, as before. By this double purchaſe, the child may be turned even in the moſt difficult caſes: but the operator, in pulling, muſt beware of over-ſtraining the ligaments of the joints.

If the legs can be extracted through the *Os externum*, let a ſingle cloth, warmed, be wrapped round them, in order to yield a

firmer

firmer hold to the accoucheur; but when they can be brought no lower than the neck of the *Uterus* or *Vagina*, he may uſe one of theſe following nooſes.

Let him take a ſtrong limber fillet or ſoft garter, half worn, about one yard and an half in length, and moderately broad and thick; if thick, an eye may be made at one end of it, by doubling about two inches and ſowing it ſtrongly; and the other end paſſed through this doubling, in order to make the nooſe, which being mounted upon the thumb and fingers of his hand, muſt be introduced, and gently ſlipped over the toes and feet of the child, ſo as to embrace the ancles; and thus applied, it muſt be drawn tight with his other hand.

If the foot or feet ſhould be ſo ſlippery, that his fingers cannot hold them, and work over the nooſe at the ſame time, it muſt be withdrawn and mounted round his hand or wriſt; with which hand, when introduced, he may take firm hold on both feet: if they are as far down as the *Vagina*, then with the fingers of his other hand he can ſlide the nooſe along the hand and fingers that hold

the

the feet, and fix it round the ancle; but if one foot and it remains within the *Uterus*, the fingers of his other hand cannot puſh up the nooſe far enough to ſlide it over the ancle, ſo that he muſt have recourſe to a director, like that for *Polypuſes*, mounted with the nooſe, which will puſh it along the hand and fingers that hold the foot. The nooſe being thus ſlipped over the fingers upon the ancle, he muſt pull the extremity of the fillet which hath paſſed the eye at the upper end of the director, and after it is cloſe drawn, bring down the inſtrument.

Some uſe a ſmall ſlender pair of forceps, to graſp the ancles and ſlide the nooſe along them; others make uſe of a fillet with a nooſe upon one end of it, fixed to an hollow tube that carries it up to be ſlipt over the ancles: and this being done, it is drawn cloſe by pulling the other end of the fillet down through the cavity of the tube: but there is ſeldom occaſion for any of theſe inſtruments, becauſe we can for the moſt part bring the feet down into the *Vagina*.

If the fillet or garter is too narrow or thin, let it be doubled in the middle, and the

nooſe

noose made by doubling the two ends through the doubling.

When the belly presents, and the head, shoulders, breech, thighs, and legs, are turned up over the back to the *Fundus uteri*; when the back presents, and all these parts are upwards; when the side presents, with the head, shoulders, breech, thighs, and legs turned to the side, back, or forepart of the *Uterus*: in all these cases, when the child is pressed into a round, or (more properly) an oval figure, it may be, for the most part, moved round, with one hand introduced into the *Uterus*, the head and shoulders pushed to the *Fundus*, and the legs and breech to the *Os internum*; which being effected, the legs are easily brought down. But these cases are more or less difficult as the feet are farther up, or lower down, because the business is to bring them downwards.

When the breast, shoulders, neck, ear, or face present to the *Os internum*, the breech, thighs, and legs being towards the *Fundus*, with the fore-parts of the *Fœtus* turned either to the side, back, or fore-part of the woman's belly; and the whole lying in a longish

longiſh form, the *Uterus* being cloſely contracted around its body like a ſheath, let the accoucheur introduce his hand into the *Vagina*, and open the *Os internum* by puſhing up the fingers and hand flattened between the parts that preſent and the inſide of the membranes; and reſt his hand in that ſituation until he can diſtinguiſh how the child lies, and form a right judgment how to turn and deliver: for, if theſe circumſtances are not maturely conſidered, he will begin to work in a confuſed manner, fatigue himſelf and the patient, and find great difficulty in turning and extracting the child.

If the feet and legs of the *Fœtus* lie towards the back, ſides, or *Fundus uteri*, the woman ought to be laid on her back, with her breech raiſed and brought a little over the bed, as formerly obſerved; becauſe in that poſition he can more eaſily reach the feet than in any other.

If they lie towards the fore-part of the *Uterus*, eſpecially when the belly is pendulous, ſhe ought to lie upon her ſide; becauſe in the other poſture it is often difficult to turn the hand up to the fore-part of the womb:

womb: whereas, if ſhe is laid on the left ſide, the right hand may be introduced at the under-part and left ſide of the brim of the *Pelvis*, where it is wideſt, and then along the fore-part of the *Uterus*, by which means the feet are more eaſily come at. If it is more convenient for the accoucheur to uſe his left hand, the patient may be turned on her right ſide. The only inconvenience attending theſe poſitions, is, that the woman cannot be kept ſo firm and ſteady, but will be apt to toſs about and ſhrink from the operator; and beſides, there may be a neceſſity for turning her upon her back, after the body is delivered, before he can extract the head, eſpecially if it be large or the *Pelvis* narrow.

The ſituation of the child being known, and the poſition of the mother adjuſted, let the proper hand be introduced, and the firſt effort always made in puſhing the preſenting part up towards the *Fundus*, either along the ſides, back, or fore-part of the *Uterus*, as is moſt convenient. If this endeavour ſucceeds, and the breech, thighs, or legs come down, the body may be delivered with eaſe: but if the head, ſhoulder, breaſt, or neck preſent, the other parts of the body being ſtretched up lengthways, and the *Uterus* ſo ſtrongly contracted around the child, that the preſenting part cannot be raiſed up, or, though puſhed upwards, immediately returns before the legs can be properly ſeized or brought down; the operator ought in that caſe to force up his hand ſlowly and gradually between the *Uterus* and the child: if the reſiſtance is great, let him reſt a little between whiles, in order to ſave the ſtrength of his hand and arm, as formerly directed, and then proceed with his efforts until he ſhall advance his hand as far as the feet; for the higher his hand is puſhed, the more will the *Uterus* be ſtretched, and the more room granted for bringing the legs along: and if, in puſhing up his hand, the fingers ſhould be intangled in the navel-ſtring or one of the arms, let him bring it a little lower, and paſs it up again on the outſide of ſuch incumbrance.

The hand being advanced as high as the *Fundus*, let him, after ſome pauſe, feel for the breech, ſlide his fingers along the thighs in ſearch of the legs and feet; of which taking hold with his whole hand, if poſſible, let him bring them down either in a ſtreight line or with an half turn: or ſhould the contraction of the *Uterus* be ſo ſtrong, that he cannot take hold of them in that manner, let him ſeize one or both ancles between his fingers, and pull them along; but if he cannot bring them down to the lower part of the *Uterus*, ſo as to apply the nooſe, he muſt try again to puſh up the body, in order ſtill more to ſtretch the *Uterus*, and obtain freer ſcope to bring them down lower: then he may apply the nooſe, and turn the child as above directed, until the head and ſhoulders are raiſed up to the *Fundus*, and the feet and breech delivered.

If one leg only can be brought down, the child being turned, and that member extracted through the *Os externum*, let the accoucheur ſlide his hand up to fetch the other; but if this cannot be done, he muſt fix a finger on the outſide of the groin of that thigh which is folded up along the belly, and bring along that buttock, as in the breech caſe, while he pulls with his other hand at the other leg; and the body being thus advanced, deliver as before directed.

When the ſhoulder preſents, and the arm lies double in the *Vagina*, let him puſh them both up; but if this cannot be done, and the hand is prevented from paſſing along, he muſt bring down the arm, and hold it with one hand, while the other is introduced; then let go and puſh up the ſhoulder, and as the child is turned, and the feet brought down, the arm will, for the moſt part, return into the *Uterus*: but if the arm that is come down be ſo much ſwelled, that it is impracticable to introduce the hand, ſo as to turn and deliver the child, he muſt ſeparate it at the joint of the ſhoulder, if it be ſo low down; or at the elbow, if he cannot reach the ſhoulder. If the limb be much mortified, it may be twiſted off; otherwiſe it may be ſnipt and ſeparated with the ſciſſars.

If the ſhoulder, by the imprudence and ignorance of the unſkilful, who pull, in expectation of delivering in that way, is forced into the *Vagina*, and part of it appears on the outſide of the *Os externum*, a vaſt force is required to return it into the *Uterus*; becauſe in this caſe, the ſhoulder, part of the ribs, breaſt, and ſide, are already pulled out of the *Uterus*, which muſt be extended ſo, as not only to receive them again, but alſo to admit the hand and arm of the accoucheur. If this diſtention cannot poſſibly be effected, he muſt ſlide his fingers to the neck of the child, and with the ſciſſars divide the head from the body; then deliver firſt the ſeparated head, or bring along the body by pulling at the arm; or, if need be, with the aſſiſtance of the crotchet: after the body is delivered, the head muſt be extracted according to the rules that will be laid down in ſect. 5.

When the forehead, face, or ear preſents, and cannot be altered with the hand into the natural poſition; or is not advanced to the *Os externum*, to aſſiſt with the forceps, the head muſt be returned, and the child delivered by the feet: but if this cannot be done, and the woman is in imminent danger, recourſe muſt be had to the crotchet.

If the navel-ſtring comes down by the child's head, and the pulſation is felt in the arteries, there is a neceſſity for turning, without

out loſs of time; for unleſs the head advances faſt, and the delivery is quick, the circulation in the veſſels will be entirely obſtructed, and the child conſequently periſh. If the head is low in the *Pelvis*, the forceps may be ſucceſsfully uſed.

No doubt, if the *Pelvis* is very narrow, or the head too large, it would be wrong to turn: in that caſe we ought to try if we can poſſibly raiſe the head, ſo as to reduce the *Funis* above it, and after that, let the labour go on; but if the waters are all gone, and a large portion of the *Funis* falls down, it is impoſſible to raiſe it, ſo as to keep it up, even although we could eaſily raiſe the head; becauſe, as one part of the *Funis* is puſhed up with the fingers, another part falls down, and evades the reduction; and to raiſe it up to the ſide, and not above the head, will be to no purpoſe: when a little only jets down at the ſide of the head, our endeavours will for the moſt part be ſucceſsful.

The antients, as well as ſome of the moderns, adviſe, in all caſes when the upper-parts, ſuch as the ſhoulders, breaſt, neck, face, or ear of the child, preſent, to puſh them upwards, and bring in the head as in the natural way; obſerving, that the *Fœtus* ought never to be delivered by the feet, except in the preſentation of the lower parts, ſuch as, the ſmall of the back, belly, ſide, breech, or legs. Were it practicable at all times to bring the head into the right poſition, a great deal of fatigue would be ſaved to the operator, much pain to the woman, and imminent danger to the child: he therefore ought to attempt this method, and may ſucceed when he is called before the membranes are broke, and feels, by the touch, that the face, ear, or any of the upper parts, preſents: in that caſe, let him open the *Os externum* ſlowly during every pain, and when the *Os internum* is ſufficiently dilated by the deſcent of the waters and membranes, let him introduce his hand into the *Uterus*, as directed in ſect. 3. betwixt the womb and the membranes, which muſt be broke; and if he finds the head ſo large, or the *Pelvis* ſo narrow, that it will be difficult to ſave the child; provided the woman is vigorous and has ſtrong pains, he may with little difficulty bring in the crown of the head, then with-

draw

draw his hand; and if the pains return and continue, the child has a good chance to be delivered alive. Even after the membranes are broke, if the preſenting part hath ſo locked up the *Os internum*, as to detain ſome portion of the waters (a circumſtance eaſily known in puſhing up the part that preſents) he muſt run up his hand ſpeedily to keep them from being diſcharged, and act in the ſame manner: but if the child is not large, nor the *Pelvis* narrow, it were pity, while his hand is in the *Uterus*, to deſiſt from turning the child and bringing it by the feet; becauſe in that caſe he may be pretty certain of ſaving it. Beſides, after the head is brought into the right poſition, ſhould the pains go off entirely (and this frequently happens) or a flooding come on, in conſequence of the force which hath been exerted, he will find great difficulty in turning after the waters have been diſcharged; for it is harder to turn when the *Vertex* preſents, than in any other poſition: whereas, in the caſe of a large head or narrow *Pelvis*, when the head is forced down by the labour-pains, and will not farther advance, the child may be ſaved by the forceps; nay, though the pains do not act ſo as to force it down, to be delivered either by the forceps or in the natural way, the head may be opened and extracted with the crotchet, which is the laſt reſource.

But this neceſſity ſeldom occurs, becauſe the caſes in which we are moſt commonly called, are after the membranes have been long broke, the waters diſcharged, and the *Uterus* ſtrongly contracted around the body of the child, which it confines, as it were, in a mould: ſo that I have frequently tried in vain to bring the head into the natural poſition; for this cannot be effected without firſt puſhing up the part that preſents, for which purpoſe great force is required; and as one hand only can be introduced, when the operator endeavours to bring in the head, the puſhing force is abated, to allow the pulling force to act; and the parts that hindered the head from preſenting are again forced down: beſides, the head is ſo large and ſlippery, that he can obtain no firm hold. He might, indeed, by introducing a finger into the mouth, lay hold on the under jaw, and bring in the face, provided the ſhoulder preſents; but

in-

inſtead of amending, this would make the caſe worſe, unleſs the child be very ſmall: yet granting the head could be brought into the natural poſition, the force neceſſarily exerted for this purpoſe would produce a flooding, which commonly weakens the patient and carries off the pains; and after all he muſt turn with leſs advantage: and if that cannot be performed when the head is brought in, he muſt have recourſe to the laſt and moſt diſagreeable method; whereas, when any other part preſents, we can always turn the child, and deliver it by the feet. This we cannot promiſe after the head is brought in; and once the operator's hand is in the *Uterus*, he ought not to run ſuch riſks.

When I firſt began to practiſe, I frequently endeavoured to adjuſt the poſition of the head in this manner, but meeting with thoſe inſupportable difficulties I have mentioned, I adhered to that method which I have always found more certain and ſafe. I have likewiſe uſed the impellens of *Albucaſis*, in order to keep up the ſhoulders or body until I could bring in the head; but the contraction was always ſo great, that the inſtrument ſlipt, and was in danger of hurting the *Uterus.* Indeed, when the ear, forehead, or the *Fontanelle* preſented, I have, by puſhing up, found the head come into the right poſition: I have likewiſe, when the forehead was towards the groin or ſide of the *Pelvis*, moved it more backwards, by which means the forceps were fixed with more eaſe; but I have much oftner failed, by the head's returning to its former ſituation.

The child is often in danger, and ſometimes loſt, when the breech preſents, and is low down in the *Pelvis*, provided the thighs are ſo ſtrongly preſſed againſt the *Funis* and belly, as to ſtop the circulation in the rope; as alſo when the child is detained by the head, after the body is delivered: in both caſes, the danger muſt be obviated by an expeditious delivery; and if the body is entangled in the navel-ſtring, it muſt be diſengaged as well as poſſible, eſpecially when the *Funis* happens to be betwixt the thighs. As I have formerly obſerved, many of theſe minute directions in laborious and præternatural caſes, may be thought idle and trifling

by

by thoſe practitioners, who without minding any ſtated rules, introduce the forceps, and taking hold on the head at random, deliver with force and violence; and who, in præternatural deliveries, thruſt up their hands into the *Uterus*, and without conſidering the poſition, ſearch for the feet, pull them down, and deliver in a hurry. Such practice may ſome times ſucceed, but will often deſtroy the child, and bruiſe and injure the parts of the mother, even to the hazard of her life.

SECT. V.

THE legs and breech of the child being brought down, and the body properly turned with the foreparts to the mother's back, let the accoucheur endeavour to bring it along; but if it is detained by the ſize of the belly, diſtended with air or water, (a caſe that frequently happens when the child has been dead for ſeveral days) let the belly be opened, by forcing into it the points of his ſciſſars: or he may tear it open with the ſharp crotchet.

The body of the child being delivered, the arms brought down, and every method hitherto

hitherto directed, unſucceſsfully uſed for the extraction of the head, which is detained by being naturally too large, over oſſified, or dropſical, or from the narrowneſs and diſtortion of the *Pelvis*; if the belly was not opened, and the child is found to be alive by the motion of the heart, or pulſation of the arteries in the *Funis*, the forceps ought to be tried; but if he finds it impracticable to deliver the head, ſo as to ſave the life of the child, he muſt, according to ſome, force the points of the ſciſſars through the lower part of the occipital bone, or through the *Foramen magnum*; then dilate the blades, ſo as to enlarge the opening, and introduce a blunt or ſharp hook. This operation rarely ſucceeds when the head is over oſſified; but may anſwer the purpoſe when the bones are ſoft and yielding, or in the caſe of an hydrocephalus: becauſe in the firſt, the aperture may ſometimes be enlarged, and in the other the water will be evacuated ſo as to diminiſh the bulk of the head, which will of conſequence come along with more eaſe.

Some recommend an inſtrument to perforate the ſcull, with double points curved and joined

joined together; which, when puſhed into the *Foramen*, are ſeparated, and take hold on the inſide; but as the opening with the ſciſſars, and introducing the blunt hook, as above, will anſwer the ſame end, it is needleſs to multiply inſtruments, eſpecially as this method is not ſo certain as the following.

If, notwithſtanding theſe endeavours, the head cannot be extracted, let the operator introduce his hand along the head, and his fingers through the *Os uteri*; then ſlide up one of the curved crotchets along the ear, betwixt his hand and the child's head, upon the upper part of which it muſt be fixed; this being done, let him withdraw his hand, take hold of the inſtrument with one hand, turning the curve of it over the forehead, and with the other, graſp the neck and ſhoulders, then pull along. The crotchet being thus fixed on the upper part, where the bones are thin and yielding, makes a large opening, through which the contents of the ſcull are emptied, the head collapſing is with more certainty extracted, and the inſtrument hath a firm hold to the laſt, at the forehead, *Os petroſum*, and baſis of the ſcull.

In introducing the crotchet, let the operator remember the caution given in chap. III. sect. 5. he must not begin to pull, until he is certain that the point of the instrument is properly fixed upon the *Vertex*; and he must keep the handle back to the *Perineum*.

The excellency of *Mesnard*'s contrivance is more conspicuous here than when the head presents; because the curvature of the crotchet allows the point to be fixed on the upper part of the scull, which is to be tore open; and in pulling, the contents are evacuated, and the head is lessened: by these means, the principal obstruction is removed; whereas the streight crotchets take so slight a hold, and slip so often, that several times I have been very much fatigued before I could effect the delivery; but have always succeeded to my satisfaction since I adopted the other kind.

If one crotchet be found insufficient, let him introduce the other in the same manner, along the opposite side, lock and join them together, and pull along, moving and turning the head, so as to humour the shape of the *Pelvis*. This method seldom fails to accomplish

complish his aim, though sometimes very great force is required; in which case, he must pull with leisure and caution.

But if all these expedients should fail, by reason of the extraordinary ossification or size of the head, or the narrowness and distortion of the *Pelvis*, after having used the crotchets without success, he must separate the body from the head with a bistory or pair of scissars; then pushing up the head into the *Uterus*, turn the face to the *Fundus* and the *Vertex* down to the *Os internum* and brim of the *Pelvis*: let him direct an assistant to press upon the woman's belly with both hands, in order to keep the *Uterus* and head firm in that position; then open the scull with the scissars, destroy the structure of the brain, and extract with the crotchets, as directed in chap. III. sect. 5.

The head is frequently left in the *Uterus* by those practitioners, who not knowing how to turn the fore-parts and face of the child towards the back-part of the *Uterus*, or how to bring it along, although it presented in that position, pull at random with all their strength; so that the neck is stretched

ſtretched and ſeparated, and the head left behind. This may alſo happen to an expert accoucheur, when the child hath been dead for many days, and the body is much mortified, even though he hath uſed all the neceſſary precautions.

In ſuch a caſe, provided the head is not very large, nor the *Pelvis* narrow, and the forehead is towards the *Sacrum*, let him ſlide up his hand along the back-part of the *Pelvis*, and introducing two fingers into the mouth, with the thumb below the chin, try to pull the forehead into the hollow of the *Sacrum*: if it ſticks at the jetting in of that bone, he muſt endeavour to move it, firſt to one ſide and then to the other. If the head is ſmall it will come along; if any fragment of the neck remains, or any part of the looſe ſkin, he may lay hold on it, and aſſiſt delivery, by pulling at it with his other hand; if the head is low down, it may be extracted with the forceps.

Should all theſe methods fail, let him puſh up his hand along the ſide of the head, until it ſhall have paſſed the *Os internum*; with the other hand let him introduce one of the

curved

curved crotchets, and fix it upon the upper part of the head; then, withdrawing the hand which was introduced, take hold on the inſtrument, and ſliding the fingers of the other hand into the mouth, he muſt pull down with both, as above directed. If the head is not over oſſified, the crotchet will tear open the ſcull; and the bulk being of conſequence diminiſhed, the whole may be brought along, even in a narrow *Pelvis*: but if it cannot be moved, even by this expedient, he muſt introduce the other crotchet along the other ſide of the head, and fixing it upon the ſcull, lock them together; then in pulling, turn the forehead down into the hollow of the *Sacrum*, and extract with an half-round turn upwards, as when delivering with the forceps.

If the forehead is towards the *Pubis*, and cannot be brought into the right poſition, let him, with his hand, puſh up the head into the *Uterus*; turn the forehead from the anterior to the ſide or back-part of it, and try to extract as before. If the child hath been dead ſome time, and is much mortified, he muſt pull cautiouſly at the under jaw;

because, ſhould that give way, he will have no other hold for pulling, or keeping the head ſteady when he attempts to extract with one crotchet.

When the head is ſo large, or the *Pelvis* ſo narrow, that none of theſe methods will ſucceed, let him puſh up, and turning the upper parts downwards, direct an aſſiſtant to preſs the patient's belly with both hands, moving them from ſide to ſide, and ſqueezing in ſuch a direction, as will force the head towards the *Os internum*, and retain it firmly in that poſition; then it muſt be opened and extracted, according to the directions given in chap. III. ſect. 7. numb. 2.

Although by theſe means I have ſucceeded in a few caſes of this kind, which have happened in my practice; yet as great difficulties may occur from inflammations of the *Pudenda*, contraction of the *Uterus*, ſlipperineſs or largeneſs of the head, and the narrowneſs of the *Pelvis*, it will not be improper to inform the reader of other methods that appear to me uſeful, particularly when the parts are much contracted and ſwelled. Let the hand be introduced into the *Vagina*,

and

and if it cannot be admitted within the *Uterus*, the fingers being inſinuated, may move the head ſo as to raiſe the face and chin to the *Fundus*, the *Vertex* being turned to the *Os internum*, and the forehead towards the ſide of the *Sacrum*. This being effected, let the operator ſlide up along one ear a blade of the long forceps, which are curved to the ſide; then change hands, and ſend up the other blade along the oppoſite ear: when they are locked, and the handles ſecured with a fillet, he muſt pull the head as low as it will come; then putting them into the hands of an aſſiſtant who will keep them in that poſition, let him make a large opening with the ſciſſars, ſqueeze the head with great force, and extract ſlowly and by degrees.

There is an old inſtrument with two ſides which turn on a pivot, formerly recommended in this caſe, and ſince improved with the addition of another ſide, by Mr. *Leveret*, who gives it the denomination of tire-tête: but as I thought the contrivance was too complex, and the blades too much confined to a circular motion, I have altered the form

 of

of it in a manner that renders it more ſimple, convenient, and leſs expenſive. Having turned down the *Vertex*, as above directed, let this inſtrument, with the three ſides joined together, be introduced along the accoucheur's hand to the upper part of the head; then let the ſides or blades be opened with the other hand, ſo as to incloſe the head, moving them circularly and lengthways in a light and eaſy manner, that they may paſs over the inequalities of the ſcalp, and avoid the reſiſtance of the head and *Uterus*: when they are exactly placed at equal diſtances from one another, let him join the handles, withdraw his hand, and tying them together with a fillet, pull down, open, and extract, as directed above; and let it be remembered, that the farther the hand can be introduced into the *Uterus*, the more eaſily will both inſtruments be managed.

When the *Pelvis* is large, or the head ſmall (in which caſes this misfortune ſeldom happens) without doubt we might ſucceed with *Mauriceau*'s broad fillet or ſling, provided it could be properly applied: but, upon trial, I found my hand ſo much cramped by the con-

contraction of the *Uterus*, and was so much incommoded by the slipperiness of the head, upon which I could not fix it so as to have sufficient hold, that after many fruitless efforts I was obliged to have recourse to the scissars and crotchets, as above.

Amand's net is attended with the same difficulties, and rather more troublesome, as it is more compounded: for when it is mounted on the operator's hand, it will be found scarce practicable to bring over the head the narrow fillet by which it is pulled along; because it commonly slides off on one side or the other.

If the *Placenta* adheres to the *Uterus*, let him first extract the head: if the cake is separated, and in his way, let him deliver it before he begins to deliver the head.

When the head is small, or the *Pelvis* large, dilating the *Foramen magnum* with the scissars, and introducing the blunt hook, may be of use either to pull the head along, or keep it down until we can fix the forceps, curve crotchet, or *Leveret*'s tire-tête.

CHAP. V.

Of TWINS.

SECT. I.

TWINS are ſuppoſed to be the effect of a double conception in one coition, when two or more *Ova* are impregnated with as many animalcula; which deſcending from the *Ovarium*, through the Fallopian tube, into the *Fundus uteri*, as they increaſe, come in contact with that part and with one another, and are ſo preſſed as to form one globular figure, and ſtretch the womb into the ſame form which it aſſumes when diſtended by one *Ovum* only; and that during the whole term of uterine geſtation, it is impoſſible to diſtinguiſh twins, either by the figure and magnitude of the *Uterus*, or by the motion of the different *Fœtuſes*: for, one child, when it is large, and ſurrounded with a great quantity of waters, will ſometimes produce as large a prominence (or even larger) in the woman's belly, than is commonly obſerved when ſhe is big with twins. One child will alſo, by moving its legs, arms, and other parts of its body, againſt different parts of the *Uterus*, at the ſame inſtant, or by intervals, yield the ſame ſenſation to the mother as may be obſerved in two or more children: for part of the motion in twins is employed on each other, as well as upon the *Uterus*.

There is therefore no certain method of diſtinguiſhing in theſe caſes, until the firſt child is delivered, and the accoucheur has examined if the *Placenta* is coming along. If this comes of itſelf, and after its extraction the mouth of the womb be felt contracted, and the operator is unwilling to give unneceſſary pain by introducing his hand into the *Uterus*; let him lay his hand upon the woman's *Abdomen*, and if nothing is left in the womb, he will generally feel it, juſt above the *Pubis*, contracted into a firm round ball, of the ſize of a child's head, or leſs: whereas, if there is another child left, the ſize will be found much larger. If the *Placenta* does not come down before the ſecond child, which is frequently the caſe, upon examining, he will commonly feel the membranes with the waters puſhed down through the *Os uteri*; or if they are broke, the head, or ſome part of the body will be felt. If, therefore, the woman has ſtrong pains, and is in no danger from floodings or weakneſs, provided the head preſents fair, and ſeems to come along, ſhe will be delivered of this alſo in the natural way.

If the membranes are not broke, if the head does not immediately follow, or if the child preſents wrong, he ought to turn and bring it immediately by the feet; in order to ſave the patient the fatigue of a ſecond labour, that may prove tedious and even dangerous, by enfeebling her too much. Beſides as the parts are fully opened by the firſt delivery, he can introduce his hand with eaſe; and as the membranes are for the moſt part whole, the waters may be kept up, and the *Fœtus* eaſily turned, as in chap. IV ſect. 2, but if the *Pelvis* is narrow, the woman ſtrong, and the head preſents, he ought to leave it to the efforts of nature.

If the firſt child preſents wrong, and in turning that, he feels another, he muſt beware

ware of breaking the membranes of one, while he is at work upon the other: but ſhould they chance to be broke, and the legs of both entanged together, (though this is ſeldom the caſe, becauſe they are commonly divided by two ſets of membranes) let the operator, when he has got hold on two legs, run up his fingers to the breech, and feel if they belong to the ſame body; and one child being delivered, let the other be turned and brought out in the ſame manner. If there are more than two, the ſame method muſt take place, in extracting one after another.

In caſe of twins, the *Placenta* of the firſt ſeldom comes along, until the ſecond child is delivered: but as this does not always happen, he ought, as formerly directed, to certify himſelf that there is nothing left in the *Uterus* when the cake comes of itſelf. Both children being delivered, let him extract both *Placentas*, if they come not of themſelves; and if they form diſtinct cakes, ſeparate firſt one, then the other; but if they are joined together, forming but one maſs, they may be delivered at once, as in chap. II. ſect. 7.

When there are three or four children, (a caſe that rarely happens) the *Placentas* are ſometimes diſtinct, and ſometimes altogether form but one round cake: but when this is macerated in water for ſome days, they, with their ſeveral membranes, may be eaſily ſeparated from one another; for they only adhere in conſequence of their long preſſure in the *Uterus*, and ſeldom have any communication of veſſels: although ſuch a communication hath lately fallen under my obſervation. *Vide* book I. chap. 3. ſect. 5.

Twins for the moſt part lie diagonally in the *Uterus*, one below the other; ſo that they ſeldom obſtruct one another at the *Os internum*.

SECT. II.

Of MONSTERS.

TWO children joined together by their bellies, (which is the moſt common caſe of monſtrous births) or by the ſides, or when the belly of the one adheres to the back of the other, having commonly but one *Funis*, are comprehended in this claſs, and ſup-

ſuppoſed to be the effect of two *Animalcula* impregnating the ſame *Ovum*; in which they grow together, and are nouriſhed by one navel-ſtring, originally belonging to the ſecundines; becauſe the veſſels pertaining to the coats of the vein and arteries, do not anaſtomoſe with the veſſels belonging to the *Fœtus*.

In ſuch a caſe, where the children were ſmall, the adheſion hath been known to ſtretch in pulling at the feet of one, ſo as to be delivered; and the other hath been afterwards brought along, in the ſame manner, without the neceſſity of a ſeparation.

When the accoucheur is called to a caſe of this kind, if the children are large, and the woman come to her full time, let him firſt attempt to deliver them by that method; but if, after the legs and part of the body of the firſt are brought down, the reſt will not follow, let him ſlide up his hand, and with his fingers examine the adheſion; then introducing the ſciſſars between his hand and the body of the *Fœtus*, endeavour to ſeparate them by ſnipping through the juncture. Should this attempt fail, he muſt diminiſh the bulk in the beſt manner he can think of, and bring the body of the firſt in different pieces, by pulling or cutting them aſunder, as he extracts with the help of the crotchet.

No certain rules can be laid down in theſe caſes, which ſeldom happen, and therefore a great deal muſt be left to the judgment and ſagacity of the operator; who muſt regulate his conduct according to the circumſtances of the caſe, and according to the directions given for delivering, when the *Pelvis* is narrow and the children extraordinary large.

Formerly, practitioners uſed ſtreight and crooked knives, with long handles, which were introduced into the *Uterus* along the hand, in order to cut and divide the bodies of children, that they might be extracted piecemeal: and this cruel practice obtained even in ſome caſes, which now we can manage with eaſe and ſafety, by turning and delivering the *Fœtus* by the feet. But, no doubt, ſome will happen in which it is impoſſible to preſerve or deliver the children without the help of inſtruments; and in ſuch an emergency, the ſciſſars are much ſafer than knives, with which the operator runs the riſk of cutting the *Uterus* or himſelf: whereas

whereas he is expoſed to no ſuch hazard from the other, which cut only betwixt the points.

SECT. III.

Of the CÆSARIAN OPERATION.

WHEN a woman cannot be delivered by any of the methods hitherto deſcribed and recommended in laborious and præternatural labours, on account of the narrowneſs or diſtortion of the *Pelvis*, into which it is ſometimes impoſſible to introduce the hand; or from large excreſcences and glandular ſwellings that fill up the *Vagina*, and cannot be removed; or from large cicatrices and adheſions in that part, and at the *Os uteri*, which cannot be ſeparated: in ſuch emergencies, if the woman is ſtrong, and of a good habit of body, the *Cæſarian* operation is certainly adviſeable, and ought to be performed; becauſe the mother and child have no other chance to be ſaved, and it is better to have recourſe to an operation which hath ſometimes ſucceeded, than leave them both to inevitable death.

Ne-

Neverthelefs, if the woman is weak, exhaufted with fruitlefs labour, violent floodings, or any other evacuation, which renders her recovery doubtful, even if fhe were delivered in the natural way: in thefe circumftances, it would be rafhnefs and prefumption to attempt an operation of this kind, which ought to be delayed until the woman expires, and then immediately performed, with a view to fave the child.

The operation hath been performed both in this and the laft century, and fometimes with fuch fuccefs, that the mother has recovered, and the child furvived. The previous fteps to be taken, are to ftrengthen the patient, if weak, with nourifhing broths and cordials; to evacuate the indurated *Fæces* with repeated glyfters; and if the bladder is diftended with urine, to draw it off with a catheter. Thefe precautions being taken, fhe muft be laid on her back, on a couch or bed, her fide on which the incifion is to be made, being raifed up by pillows placed below the fame: the operation may be performed on either fide, though the left is commonly preferred to the right; becaufe in this

this laſt the liver extends lower. The apparatus conſiſts of a biſtory, probe, ſciſſars, large needles threaded, ſpunges, warm water, pledgets, a large tent or doſſil, compreſſes, and a bandage for the belly.

If the weather is cold, the patient muſt be kept warm, and no part of the belly uncovered, except that on which the inciſion is to be made: if the operator be a young practitioner, the place may be marked by drawing a line along the middle ſpace between the navel and the *Os ilium*, about ſix or ſeven inches in length, ſlanting forwards towards the left groin, and beginning as high as the navel.

According to this direction, let him hold the ſkin of the *Abdomen* tenſe between the finger and thumb of one hand, and with the biſtory in the other, make a longitudinal inciſion through the *Cutis* to the *Membrana adipoſa*, which, with the muſcles, muſt be ſlowly diſſected and ſeparated, until he reaches the *Peritonæum*, which muſt be divided very cautiouſly, for fear of wounding the inteſtines that frequently ſtart up at the ſides, eſpecially if the membranes are broke,

the

the waters diſcharged, and the *Uterus* contracted.

The *Peritoneum* being laid bare, it may either be pinched up by the fingers, or ſlowly diſſected with the biſtory, until an opening is made ſufficient to admit the fore-finger, which muſt be introduced as a director for the biſtory or ſciſſars in making an effectual dilatation. If the inteſtines puſh out, let them be preſſed downwards, ſo as that the *Uterus* may come in contact with the opening. If the womb is ſtill diſtended with the waters, and at ſome diſtance from the child, the operator may make upon it a longitudinal inciſion at once; but if it is contracted cloſe round the body of the *Fœtus*, he muſt pinch it up, and dilate in the ſame cautious manner practiſed upon the *Peritoneum*, taking care to avoid wounding the Fallopian tubes, ligaments, and bladder: then introducing his hand, he may take out the child and ſecundines. If the woman is ſtrong, the *Uterus* immediately contracts, ſo as that the opening, which at firſt extended to about ſix or ſeven inches, is reduced to two, or leſs; and in conſequence of this contraction, the veſſels

being

being ſhrunk up, a great effuſion of blood is prevented.

The coagulated blood being removed, and what is ſtill fluid ſpunged up, the inciſion in the *Abdomen* muſt be ſtitched with the interrupted *Suture*, and ſufficient room left between the laſt ſtitch and the lower end of the opening, for the diſcharge of the moiſture and extravaſated fluid. The wound may be dreſſed with dry pledgets or doſſils dipped in ſome liquid balſam warmed, covered with compreſſes moiſtened with wine, and a bandage to keep on the dreſſings and ſuſtain the belly. Some authors obſerve, that the *Cutis* and muſcles only ſhould be taken up in the *Suture*, leſt bad ſymptoms ſhould ariſe from ſtitching the *Peritoneum*.

The woman muſt be kept in bed as quiet as poſſible, and every thing adminiſtred to promote the *Lochia*, perſpiration, and ſleep; which will prevent a fever, and other dangerous ſymptoms. If ſhe hath loſt a great quantity of blood from the wounds in the *Uterus* and *Abdomen*, ſo as to be in danger from innition, broths, caudles, and wine,

ought

ought to be given in ſmall quantities, and frequently repeated. The *Cort. peruvian.* adminiſtred in powder, decoction, or extract, is frequently of great ſervice in this caſe: and for farther information on this ſubject, the reader may conſult *Ruſſetus*, the memoirs of the academy of ſurgeons at *Paris*, and *Heiſter*'s ſurgery.

BOOK

BOOK IV.

CHAP. I.

Of the Management of Women from the Time of their Delivery to the End of the Month, with the ſeveral Diſeaſes to which they are ſubject during that Period.

SECT. I.

Of the EXTERNAL APPLICATION.

THE woman being delivered of the child and *Placenta*, let a ſoft linnen cloth, warmed, be applied to the external parts; and if ſhe complains much of a ſmarting ſoreneſs, ſome pomatum may be ſpread upon it. The linnen that was laid below her, to ſpunge up the diſcharges, muſt be removed, and replaced with others that

are

are clean, dry, and warm. Let her lie on her back, with her legs extended cloſe to each other; or upon her ſide, if ſhe thinks ſhe can lie eaſier in that poſition, until ſhe recovers from the fatigue: if ſhe is ſpent and exhauſted, let her take a little warm wine or caudle, or, according to the common cuſtom, ſome nutmeg and ſugar grated together in a ſpoon: the principal deſign of adminiſtring this cordial, which among the good women is ſeldom neglected, is to ſupply the want of ſome cordial draught, when the patient is too weak to be raiſed, or ſuppoſed to be in danger of reachings from her ſtomach's being over-loaded. When ſhe hath, in ſome meaſure, recovered her ſtrength and ſpirits, let the cloaths be removed from the parts, and others applied in their room; and if there is a large diſcharge from the *Uterus*, let the wet linnen below her be alſo ſhifted, that ſhe may not run the riſque of catching cold.

When the patient is either weak or faintiſh, ſhe ought not to be taken out of bed, or even raiſed up to have her head and body ſhifted, until

until ſhe is a little recruited; otherwiſe ſhe will be in danger of repeated faintings, attended with convulſions, which ſometimes end in death. To prevent theſe bad conſequences, her ſkirt and petticoats ought to be looſened and pulled down over the legs, and replaced by another well warmed, with a broad head-band to be ſlipt in below, and brought up over her thighs and hips: a warm double cloth muſt be laid on the belly, which is to be ſurrounded by the head-band of the ſkirt pinned moderately tight over the cloth, in order to compreſs the *Viſcera* and the relaxed *Parietes* of the *Abdomen*, more or leſs, as the woman can eaſily bear it; by which means, the *Uterus* is kept firm in the lower part of the *Abdomen*, and prevented from rolling from ſide to ſide, when the patient is turned: but the principal end of this compreſſion, is to hinder too great a quantity of blood from ruſhing into the relaxed veſſels of the *Abdominal* contents; eſpecially when the *Uterus* is emptied all of a ſudden, by a quick delivery. The preſſure being thus ſuddenly removed, the head is all at once robbed of its proportion of blood, and the

 im-

immediate revulsion precipitates the patient into dangerous *Lypothymias*.

For this reason, the belly ought to be firmly compressed by the hands of an assistant, until the bandage is applied; or, in lieu of it, a long towel, sheet, or roller, to make a suitable compression: but, for this purpose, different methods are used in different countries, or according to the different circumstances of the patients. The head-cloaths and shift ought also to be changed, because with sweating in time of labour, they are rendered wet and disagreeable. Several other applications are necessary, when the external or internal parts are rent or inflamed, misfortunes that sometimes happen in laborious and præternatural cases.

The directions for ordering the bed in time of labour, and of the applications after delivery, are absolutely necessary to be known by young practitioners; because all these directions are for the ease and safety of the patient, when attended by unexperienced nurses.

Numb. I.

Inflammations of the *Labia pudendi*, *Rectum*, *Urethra*, *Vagina*, and *Uterus*, chiefly happen when the head, ſhoulder, breech, or any other part of the *Fœtus*, hath been forced into the *Pelvis*, and long retained in that ſituation; ſo that by many and ſtrong pains, the delivery was effected, or great force and violence were required to turn or extract the child. Theſe inflammations, if ſlight, are commonly relieved, or altogether reſolved, by a plentiful diſcharge of the *Lochia*, reſt, and profuſe ſweating; but if violent, blooding, warm fomentations, cataplaſms, and emollient glyſters, may be neceſſary; though the firſt and laſt muſt be uſed with caution.

If the preſſure hath been ſo great, as totally to obſtruct the circulating fluids in thoſe parts, a mortification enſues; either total, by which the woman is ſoon deſtroyed, or partial, when the mortified parts ſeparate and caſt off in thick ſloughs, then digeſt and are healed as a common ſore, provided the patient be of a good habit of body: but if the oppoſite parts are alſo affected in the ſame manner, and both ſides preſſed together; as for example, in the *Uterus*, *Os internum*, *Vagina*, or *Os externum*, or if the internal membrane of the whole inner ſurface ſloughs off, then there is danger of a coaleſcence or growing together, by which are formed callosities; and theſe, if they happen in the *Os internum*, *Vagina*, or *Os externum*, will produce difficult and dangerous labours in the next parturition; and if in the *Uterus*, will altogether prevent conception, though this rarely happens, becauſe of the continual draining of the moiſture that is diſcharged from the womb. In order to avoid this miſchance, emollient injections ought frequently to be thrown up into the *Uterus*, and large tents or doſſils, dipt in vulnerary balſams, applied in the *Vagina* and *Os externum*.

NUMB. II.

IF in conſequence of the long preſſure of the child's head, at that part of the *Vagina* where its outward ſurface is attached to the back and under part of the bladder, the mortification affects the coats of the *Veſica urina-*

ria,

ria, as well as thoſe of the *Vagina*, when the ſloughs falls off, the urine will paſs that way, and hinder the opening (if large) from being cloſed; this is an inexpreſſible inconvenience and misfortune to the poor woman, both from the ſmell and continual wetting of her cloaths. The *Vagina* and bladder may alſo be lacerated by the forceps, crotchet, or any other inſtrument imprudently forced up; but, in that caſe, the urine is immediately diſcharged through the wound; whereas, in a mortification, it comes in a natural way, until the ſlough begins to ſeparate and fall off.

As ſoon as this misfortune is known, the cure ought to be attempted: this (according to ſome) conſiſts in keeping a flexible catheter always in the bladder, that the urine may be continually ſolicited to come through the *Urethra*, rather than through the *Vagina*; bul if this precaution hath been neglected, and the lips of the ulcer are turned callous, we are directed to pare them off with a curve knife, buttoned at the point, or conſume them with lunar cauſtick; and if the opening is large, to cloſe it with a double ſtitch, keeping the flexible catheter in the bladder until it is entirely filled up: but, I wiſh this operation may not be found impracticable.

NUMB. III.

THE *Os externum* is frequently tore, particularly at the *Perinæum*; and ſometimes the laceration reaches to the *Anus*. At other times (but more ſeldom) both *Vagina* and *Rectum* are tore for the ſpace of two or three inches upwards, and the two form but one cavity at the lower part. This laceration is frequently occaſioned from the exceſſive largeneſs of the child's head; from the rigidity of the fibres in women, who are near the borders of forty when their firſt children are born; from the accoucheur's neglecting to ſlide the *Perinæum* over the head, when it is forcibly propelled by the pains, or from his omitting to keep up the head with the flat of his hand, that it may not come too ſuddenly along; from too great violence uſed in laborious or præternatural labours; and from the operator's incautious manner of thruſting in his hand. If the laceration be ſmall, the part ſoon heals up, and the only inconvenience attending the wound, is a ſmarting after making water; and when the laceration is large, extending to the edge of the *Sphincter ani*, or even farther, this pain is ſtill more troubleſome, and increaſed upon the leaſt motion, by the friction of the lips againſt each other. This diſagreeable rubbing, is (according to ſome writers) prevented by making two deep ſtitches that will keep the lips together: but in this caſe, we can ſeldom cure by the firſt intention, on account of the moiſture that is continually paſſing that way; namely, the *Lochia* and urine, that inſinuate themſelves into the wound. Beſides, the lips are tore and ragged, and the hold we have is but ſlender.

In the third caſe, it is ſuppoſed, that there is an abſolute neceſſity to make, as ſoon as poſſible, two, three, or ſometimes four deep ſtitches through the tore *Vagina* and *Rectum*, the knots being tied in the *Vagina*, and two more ſtitches in the *Perinæum*, to aſſiſt the re-union of the parts: for, if the *Sphincter ani* is entirely ſeparated, and continues in that condition, the patient can ſeldom retain her excrements for any length of time. If this mis-

misfortune ſhould remain unknown, or the operation unperformed, on account of the woman's weakneſs, until the lips of the wound are grown callous, theſe callous edges muſt be pared off with ſciſſars; or if that ſhould be found impracticable, ſcarified with the point of a lancet or biſtory, and then ſtitched, as above directed: and the ſtitches muſt be made very deep, otherwiſe they will not hold; becauſe there is but little muſcular fleſh in the *Vagina* and *Rectum*: bnt the *Colon* ought firſt to be emptied with glyſters, and the patient take little or no ſolid food, that the ſtitches may not be overſtrained when ſhe goes to ſtool. When the laceration reaches ſo high, as to endanger the woman's retentive faculty, this method, doubtleſs, ought to be tried; but not otherwiſe, becauſe the operation very rarely ſucceeds.

When the *Os internum* is tore from the ſame cauſes, all that can be done, is to keep the patient ſtrictly to the regimen we have directed for women after delivery, and take care that ſhe ſhall move as little as poſſible during the firſt three weeks.

The

The rents or lacerations that happen to the *Uterus*, are of more dangerous conſequence, and, indeed, commonly accounted mortal; therefore they demand the utmoſt care and circumſpection, in all the different caſes. If the patient is plethoric, ſhe ought to be blooded, in order to prevent a fever, unleſs ſhe hath undergone a conſiderable diſcharge from the *Uterus*; ſhe ought to be kept very quiet and motionleſs, to take nothing but ſpoon-meat, and even of that, a little at a time; drink diluting liquors, ſuch as, barley-water, and very weak broths.

SECT. II.

Of Air, Diet, Sleeping, and Watching, Motion and Reſt, Retention and Excretion, and the Paſſions of the Mind.

ALthough we cannot remove the patient immediately after delivery into another climate, we can qualify the air, ſo as to keep it in a moderate and ſalutary temper, by rendering it warm or cold, moiſt or dry, according to the circumſtances of the occaſion.

With

With regard to diet, women in time of labour, and even till the ninth day after delivery, ought to eat little ſolid food, and none at all during the firſt five or ſeven: let them drink plentifully of warm, diluting fluids, ſuch as, barley-water, gruel, chicken-water, and teas; caudles are alſo commonly uſed, compoſed of water-gruel boiled up with mace and cinnamon, to which, when ſtrained, is added a third or fourth part of white wine, or leſs, if the patient drinks plentifully, ſweetened with ſugar to their taſte: this compoſition is termed white caudle; whereas, if ale is uſed inſtead of wine, it goes under the name of brown caudle. In ſome countries, eggs are added to both kinds; but in that caſe, the woman is not permitted to eat meat or broths till after the fifth or ſeventh day: in this country, however, as eggs are no part of the ingredients, the patient is indulged with weak broth ſooner, and ſometimes allowed to eat a little boiled chicken. But all theſe different preparations are to be preſcribed weaker or ſtronger, with regard to the ſpices, wine, or ale, according to the different conſtitutions and ſituations of dif-

different patients: fc. example; if ſhe is low and weak, in conſequence of an extraordinary diſcharge of any kind, either before or after delivery; or if the weather is cold, the caudles and broths may be made the ſtronger: but if ſhe is of a full habit of body, and has the leaſt tendency to a fever, or if the ſeaſon is exceſſively hot, theſe drinks ought to be of a very weak conſiſtence; or the patient reſtricted to gruel, tea, barley, and chicken-water, and theſe varied according to the emergency of the caſe.

Her food muſt be light and eaſy of digeſtion, ſuch as panada, biſcuit, and ſago: about the fifth or ſeventh day ſhe may eat a little boiled chicken, or the lighteſt kind of young meat: but theſe laſt may be given ſooner or later, according to the circumſtance of the caſe, and the appetite of the patient. In the regimen as to eating and drinking, we ſhould rather err on the abſtemious ſide, than indulge the woman with meat and ſtrong fermented liquors, even if theſe laſt ſhould be moſt agreeable to her palate: for we find by experience, that they are apt to increaſe or bring on fevers, and that the moſt nouriſhing

riſhing and ſalutary diet, is that which we have above preſcribed. Every thing that is difficult of digeſtion, or quickens the circulating fluids, muſt of neceſſity promote a fever; by which, the neceſſary diſcharges are obſtructed, and the patient's life endangered.

As to the article of ſleeping and watching, the patient muſt be kept as free from noiſe as poſſible, by covering the floors and ſtairs with carpets and cloths, oiling the hinges of the doors, ſilencing the bells, tying up the knockers, and in noiſy ſtreets ſtrowing the pavement with ſtraw: if, notwithſtanding theſe precautions, ſhe is diſturbed, her ears muſt be ſtuffed with cotton, and opiates adminiſtred to procure ſleep; becauſe watching makes her reſtleſs, prevents perſpiration, and promotes a fever.

Motion and reſt are another part of the nonnaturals, to which we ought to pay particular regard. By toſſing about, getting out of bed, or ſitting up too long, the perſpiration is diſcouraged and interrupted; and in this laſt attitude, the *Uterus*, not yet fully contracted, hangs down, ſtretching the ligaments, occaſioning pain, cold ſhiverings, and a fever: for the prevention of theſe bad ſymptoms, the patient muſt be kept quiet in bed till after the fourth or fifth day, and then to be gently lifted up in the bed-cloaths, in a lying poſture, until the bed can be adjuſted, into which ſhe muſt be immediately reconveyed, there to continue, for the moſt part, till the ninth day; after which period, women are not ſo ſubject to fevers, as immediately after delivery. Some there are, who from the nature of their conſtitutions, or other accidents, recover more ſlowly; and ſuch are to be treated with the ſame caution after, as before, the ninth day, as the caſe ſeems to indicate: others get up, walk about, and recover, in a much ſhorter time; but theſe may, ſome time or other, pay dearly for their foolhardineſs, by encouraging dangerous fevers: ſo that we ought rather to err on the ſafe ſide, than run any riſque whatſoever.

What next comes under conſideration, is the circumſtance of retention and excretion. We have formerly obſerved, that in time of labour, before the head of the child is locked into the *Pelvis*, if the woman has not had

eaſy

easy passage in her belly that same day, the *Rectum* and *Colon* ought to be emptied by a glyster; which will assist the labour, prevent the disagreeable excretion of the *Fæces* before the child's head, and enable the patient to remain two or three days after, without the necessity of going to stool. However, should this precaution be neglected, and the patient very costive after delivery, we must beware of throwing up stimulating glysters, or administring strong catharticks, lest they should bring on too many loose stools; which, if they cannot be stopt, sometimes produce fatal consequences, by obstructing the perspiration and *Lochia*, and exhausting the woman, so as that she will die all of a sudden; a catastrophe which hath frequently happened from this practice. Wherefore, if it be necessary to empty the intestines, we ought to prescribe nothing but emollient glysters, or some very gentle opener, such as manna, or *Elect. Lenitivum*: for the retention of urine that sometimes happens after labour, we have already proposed a remedy in book II. chap. 2. and sect. 3. But no excretion is of more consequence to the patient's recovery, than

than a ſree perſpiration; which is ſo abſolutely neceſſary, that unleſs ſhe has a moiſture continually on the ſurface of her body, for ſome days after the birth, ſhe ſeldom recovers to advantage: her health, therefore, in a great meaſure depends upon her enjoying undiſturbed repoſe, and a conſtant breathing ſweat, which prevents a fever, by carrying off the tenſion, and aſſiſts the equal diſcharge of the *Lochia*: and when theſe are obſtructed, and a fever enſues with pain and reſtleſsneſs, nothing relieves the patient ſo effectually as reſt and profuſe ſweating, procured by opiates and ſudorificks at the beginning of the complaints; yet theſe laſt muſt be more cautiouſly preſcribed in exceſſive hot, than in cool weather.

The laſt of the nonnaturals to be conſidered, are the paſſions of the mind, which alſo require particular attention. The patient's imagination muſt not be diſturbed by the news of any extraordinary accident which may have happened to her family or friends: for ſuch information hath been known to carry off the labour-pains intirely, after they were begun, and the woman has ſunk under her dejection of ſpirits; and even after delivery, theſe unſeaſonable communications have produced ſuch anxiety as obſtructed all the neceſſary excretions, and brought on a violent fever and convulſions, that ended in death.

SECT. III.

Of violent FLOODINGS.

ALL women, when the *Placenta* ſeparates, and after it is delivered, loſe more or leſs red blood, from the quantity of half a pound, to that of one pound, or even two; but ſhould it exceed this proportion, and continue to flow without diminution, the patient is in great danger of her life: this hazardous hæmorrhage is known by the violence of the diſcharge, wetting freſh cloths as faſt as they can be applied; from the pulſe becoming low and weak, and the countenance turning pale; then the extremities grow cold, ſhe ſinks into faintings, and, if the diſcharge is not ſpeedily ſtopt, or diminiſhed, is ſeized with convulſions, which often terminate in death.

This dangerous efflux is occaſioned by every thing that hinders the emptied *Uterus* from

from contracting, ſuch as, great weakneſs and laſſitude, in conſequence of repeated floodings before delivery; the ſudden evacuation of the *Uterus*; ſometimes, though ſeldom, it proceeds from part of the *Placenta*'s being left in the womb: it may happen when there is another child, or more, ſtill undelivered; when the womb is kept diſtended with a large quantity of coagulated blood; or when it is inverted by pulling too forcibly at the *Placenta*. *Vide* book II. chap. 3. ſect. 3.

In this caſe, as there is no time to be loſt, and internal medicines cannot act ſo ſuddenly as to anſwer the purpoſe, we muſt have immediate recourſe to external application. If the diſorder be owing to weakneſs, by which the *Uterus* is diſabled from contracting itſelf, ſo that the mouths of the veſſels are left open; or, though contracted a little, yet not enough to reſtrain the hæmorrhage of the thin blood; or if, in ſeparating the *Placenta*, the accoucheur has ſcratched or tore the inner ſurface or membrane of the womb; in theſe caſes, ſuch things muſt be uſed as will aſſiſt the contractile power of the *Uterus*, and hinder the blood from flowing ſo faſt into it and the neighbouring veſſels: for this purpoſe, cloths dipped in any cold reſtringent fluid, ſuch as oxycrate, or red tart wine, may be applied to the back and belly. Some preſcribe venæſection in the arm, to the amount of five or ſix ounces, with a view of making revulſion: if the pulſe is ſtrong, this may be proper; otherwiſe, it will do more harm than good: others order ligatures, for compreſſing the returning veins at the hams, arms, and neck, to retain as much blood as poſſible in the extremities and head. Beſides theſe applications, the *Vagina* may be filled with tow or linnen rags, dipped in the above mentioned liquids, in which a little allum, or *Sacchar-ſaturni* hath been diſſolved: nay, ſome practitioners inject proof ſpirits warmed, or, ſoaking them up in a rag or ſpunge, introduce and ſqueeze them in the *Uterus*, in order to conſtringe the veſſels.

If the flooding proceeds from another child, the retention of the *Placenta*, or coagulated blood, theſe ought immediately to be extracted, and if there is an inverſion of the *Uterus*, it muſt be ſpeedily reduced. Should the hæmorrhage, by theſe methods, abate a little, but ſtill continue to flow, though not in ſuch a quantity as to bring on ſudden death, ſome red wine and jelly ought to be preſcribed for the patient, who ſhould take it frequently, and a little at a time; but above all things, chicken or mutton broths, adminiſtred in the ſame manner, for fear of overloading the weakened ſtomach, and occaſioning reachings: theſe repeated in ſmall quantities, will gradually fill the exhauſted veſſels, and keep up the circulation. If the pulſe continues ſtrong, it will be proper to order repeated draughts of barley-water, acidulated with *Elixir vitrioli*: but if the circulation be weak and languid, extract of the bark diſſolved in *Aq. cinnamomitenuis*, and given in ſmall draughts, or exhibited in any other form, will be ſerviceable; at the ſame time, lulling the patient to reſt with opiates. Theſe, indeed, when the firſt violence of the flood is abated, if properly and cautiouſly uſed, are generally more effectual than any other medicine.

SECT. IV.

Of the AFTER-PAINS.

AFter-pains commonly happen when the fibrous part of the blood is retained in the *Uterus* or *Vagina*, and formed into large clots, which are detained by the ſudden contraction of the *Os internum* and *Externum*, after the *Placenta* is delivered: or, if theſe ſhould be extracted, others will ſometimes be formed, though not ſo large as the firſt, becauſe the cavity of the womb is continually diminiſhing after the birth. The *Uterus*, in contracting, preſſes down theſe coagulums to the *Os internum*; which being again gradually ſtretched, produces a degree of labour-pains, owing to the irritation of its nerves: in conſequence of this uneaſineſs, the woman ſqueezes the womb as in real labour; the force being increaſed, the clots are puſhed along, and when they are delivered, ſhe grows eaſy. The larger the quantity is of this coagulated blood, the ſeverer are the pains, and the longer they continue.

Women in the firſt child, ſeldom have after-pains; becauſe, after delivery, the womb is ſuppoſed to contract, and puſh off the clots with greater force in the firſt, than in the following labours: after-pains may alſo proceed from obſtructions in the veſſels, and irritations at the *Os internum*. In order to prevent or remove theſe pains, as ſoon as the *Placenta* is ſeparated and delivered, the hand being introduced into the *Uterus*, may clear it of all the *Coagula*. When the womb is felt through the *Parietes* of the *Abdomen* larger than uſual, it may be taken for granted, that there is either another child, or a large quantity of this clotted blood; and which ſoever it may be, there is a neceſſity for its being extracted. If the *Placenta* comes away of itſelf, and the after-pains are violent, they may be alleviated and carried off by an opiate: for, by ſleeping and ſweating plentifully, the irritation is removed, the evacuations are increaſed, the *Os uteri* is inſenſibly relaxed, and the *Coagula* ſlide eaſily along. When the diſcharge of the *Lochia* is ſmall, the after-pains, if moderate, ought not to be reſtrained; becauſe the ſqueezing which they occaſion, promotes the other evacuation, which is neceſſary for the recovery of the patient. After-pains may alſo proceed from an obſtruction in ſome of the veſſels, occaſioning a ſmall inflammation of the *Os internum* and ligaments; and the ſqueezing thereby occaſioned, may not only help to propel the obſtructing fluid, but alſo (if not too violent) contribute to the natural diſcharges.

SECT. V.

Of the LOCHIA.

WE have already obſerved, that the delivery of the child and *Placenta* is followed by an efflux of more or leſs blood, diſcharged from the *Uterus*; which, by the immediate evacuation of the large veſſels, is allowed to contract itſelf the more freely, without the danger of an inflammation, which would probably happen in the contraction, if the great veſſels were not emptied at the ſame time: but as the fluids in the ſmaller veſſels cannot be ſo ſoon evacuated, or returned into the *Vena cava*, it is neceſſary, that after the great diſcharge is abated, a ſlow and gradual evacuation ſhould continue, until the womb

ſhall

ſhall be contracted to near the ſame ſize which it had before pregnancy; and to this it attains about the eighteenth or twentieth day after delivery, though the period is different in different women.

When the large veſſels are emptied immediately after delivery, the diſcharge frequently ceaſes for ſeveral hours, until the fluids in the ſmaller veſſels are propelled into the larger, and then begins to flow again, of a paler colour.

The red colour of the *Lochia* commonly continues till the fifth day, though it is always turning more and more ſerous from the beginning; but about the fifth day, it flows of a clear, or ſometimes (though ſeldom) of a greeniſh tint: for, the mouths of the veſſels growing gradually narrower, by the contraction of the *Uterus*, at laſt, allow the ſerous part only to paſs: as for the greeniſh hue, it is ſuppoſed to proceed from a diſſolution of the cellular or cribriform membrane or *Mucus*, that ſurrounded the ſurface of the *Placenta* and *Chorion*; part of which being left in the *Uterus*, becomes livid, decays, and, dif-diſſolving, mixes with and tinctures the diſcharge as it paſſes along.

Though the *Lochia*, as we have already obſerved, commonly continue to the eighteenth or twentieth day, they are every day diminiſhing in quantity, and ſooneſt ceaſe in thoſe women who ſuckle their children, or have had an extraordinary diſcharge at firſt; but the colour, quantity, and duration, differ in different women: in ſome patients, the red colour diſappears on the firſt or ſecond day; and in others, though rarely, it continues more or leſs to the end of the month: the evacuation in ſome is very ſmall, in others exceſſive; in one woman it ceaſes very ſoon, in another flows during the whole month: yet all of theſe patients ſhall do well.

Some alledge, that this diſcharge from the *Uterus*, is the ſame with that from a wound of a large ſurface; but it is more reaſonable to ſuppoſe, that the change of colour and diminution of quantity, proceeds from the ſlow contraction of the veſſels: becauſe, previous to *Pus*, there muſt have been lacerations or impoſthumes, and in women who have ſuddenly died after delivery, no wound or ex-

coriation

coriation hath appeared upon the inner ſurface of the womb, which is ſometimes found altogether ſmooth, and at other times rough and unequal on that part to which the *Placenta* adhered. The ſpace that this occupied before delivery, from being ſix inches in diameter, or eighteeen inches in circumference, will ſoon after the birth, be contracted to one third or fourth of theſe dimenſions.

SECT. VI.

Of the MILK FEVER.

ABOUT the fourth day, the breaſts generally begin to grow turgid and painful. We have formerly obſerved, that during the time of uterine geſtation, the breaſts in moſt women gradually increaſe till the delivery, growing ſofter as they are enlarged by the veſſels being more and more filled with fluids; and by this gradual diſtention, they are prepared for ſecreting the milk from the blood, after delivery. During the two or three firſt days after parturition, eſpecially when the woman has undergone a large diſcharge,

charge, the breaſts have been ſometimes obſerved to ſubſide and grow flaccid; and about the third or fourth day, when the *Lochia* begin to decreaſe, the breaſts ſwell again to their former ſize, and ſtretch more and more, until the milk, being ſecreted, is either ſucked by the child, or frequently of itſelf runs out at the nipples.

Moſt of the complaints incident to women after delivery, proceed either from the obſtruction of the *Lochia* in the *Uterus*, or of the milk in the breaſts, occaſioned by any thing that will produce a fever; ſuch as catching cold, long and ſevere labour, eating food that is hard of digeſtion, and drinking fluids that quicken the circulation of the blood in the large veſſels; by which means, the ſmaller, with all the ſecretory and excretory ducts, are obſtructed.

The diſcharge of the *Lochia* being ſo different in women of different conſtitutions, and beſides, in ſome meaſure depending upon the method of management, and the way of life peculiar to the patient, we are not to judge of her ſituation from the colour, quantity, and duration of them, but from the other

other ſymptoms that attend the diſcharge; and if the woman ſeems hearty, and in a fair way of recovery, nothing ought to be done with a view to augment or diminiſh the evacuation. If the diſcharge be greater than ſhe can bear, it will be attended with all the ſymptoms of inanition; but as the *Lochia* ſeldom flow ſo violently, as to deſtroy the patient of a ſudden, ſhe may be ſupported by a proper, nouriſhing diet, aſſiſted with cordial and reſtorative medicines. Let her, for example, uſe broths, gellies, and aſſes milk; if the pulſe is languid and ſunk, ſhe may take repeated doſes of the *Confect. Cardiac*, with mixtures compoſed of the cordial waters and volatile ſpirits: Subaſtringents and opiates frequently adminiſtred, with the *Cort. Peruvian.* in different forms, and auſtere wines, are of great ſervice. On the other hand, when the diſcharge is too ſmall, or hath ceaſed altogether, the ſymptoms are more dangerous, and require the contrary method of cure: for, now the buſineſs is to remove a too great plenitude of the veſſels in and about the *Uterus*, occaſioning tenſion, pain, and labour, in the circulating fluids; from

from whence proceed great heat in the part, reſtleſsneſs, fever, a full, hard, quick pulſe, pains in the head and back, nauſea, and difficulty of breathing. Theſe complaints, if not at firſt prevented, or removed by reſt and plentiful ſweating, muſt be treated with venæſection and the antiphlogiſtic method.

When the obſtruction is recent, let the patient lie quiet, and encourage a plentiful diaphoreſis, by drinking frequently of warm, weak, diluting fluids, ſuch as water-gruel, barley water, tea, or weak chicken broth: ſhe may likewiſe take opiates and ſudorificks in different forms, as may be agreeable to her ſtomach. *Theriac. Androm.* from ʒß. to ʒ1. *Laud. liquid.* from gut. x to gut. xx. *Pilul. Saponac.* from gr. v. to gr. x. or *Syr. de Meconio.* from ℥ß. to ℥i. Theſe may be repeated occaſionally, with other forms of opiates; and if they fail to procure reſt and ſweating, the following diaphoretics, without opium, ought to be adminiſtred.

℞ *Pulv. Contrayerv. Com.* ʒß. *Pulv. Caſtor. Ruſſ. Sal. ſuccin.* āā gr. v. *Syr. Croci* q. ſ. f. *Bolus ſtatim ſumendus cum hauſt. ſequent. et*

re-

repetat. quarta vel ſexta quaque hora ad tres vices vel ut opus fuerit.

℞ *Aq. Cinnamom.* ten ℥iß. *cum ſpiritu. Syr. croci āā* ʒij. *adde Sal. vol.* C. C. gr. iv. m.

Should theſe methods be uſed without ſucceſs, and the patient far from being relieved by reſt, plentiful ſweating, or a ſufficient diſcharge of the obſtructed *Lochia*, labour under an hot, dry ſkin, anxiety, and a quick, hard, and full pulſe, the warm diaphoretics muſt be laid aſide; becauſe if they fail of having the deſired effect, they muſt neceſſarily increaſe the fever and obſtruction, and recourſe be had to bleeding at the arm or ancle, to more or leſs quantity, according to the degree of fever and obſtruction; and this evacuation muſt be repeated as there is occaſion: When the obſtruction is not total, it is ſuppoſed more proper to bleed at the ancle than at the arm; and at this laſt, when the diſcharge is altogether ſtopped. Her ordinary drink ought to be impregnated with nitre, and the following draughts, or others of the ſame kind, preſcribed.

℞ *Sal. Abſynth.* ℈i. *Succ. Limon.* ℥ß. *Aq. Cinnamom. ſimp.* ℥iß. *Pulv. contrayerv. comp.*

comp. ℈i. *Sacch. Alb.* q. ſ. f. *Hauſtus ſtatim ſumendus, et quarta vel ſexta quaque hora repetendus.*

If ſhe is coſtive, emollient and gently-opening glyſters may be occaſionally injected; and her breaſts muſt be fomented and ſucked, either by the mouth or pipe-glaſſes. If, by theſe means, the fever is abated, and the neceſſary diſcharges return, the patient commonly recovers; but, if the complaints continue, the antiphlogiſtic method muſt ſtill be purſued. If, notwithſtanding theſe efforts, the fever is not diminiſhed or removed by a plentiful diſcharge of the *Lochia* from the *Uterus*, the milk from the breaſts, or by a critical evacuation by ſweat, urine, or ſtool, and the woman is every now and then attacked with cold ſhiverings, an abſceſs or abſceſſes will probably be formed in the *Uterus* or neighbouring parts, or in the breaſts; and ſometimes the matter will be tranſlated to other ſituations, and the ſeat of it foretold from the part's being affected with violent pains: theſe abſceſſes are more or leſs dangerous, according to the place in which they hap-

happen, the largeneſs of the ſuppuration, and the good or bad conſtitution of the patient.

If, when the pains in the epigaſtric region are violent, and the fever increaſed to a very high degree, the patient ſhould all of a ſudden enjoy a ceſſation from pain, without any previous diſcharge, or critical eruption, the phyſician may pronounce that a mortification is begun; eſpecially if, at the ſame time, the pulſe becomes low, quick, wavering, and intermitting; if the woman's countenance, from being florid, turns duſky and pale, while ſhe herſelf, and all the attendants, conceive her much mended; in that caſe, ſhe will grow delirious, and die in a very ſhort time.

What we have ſaid on this ſubject, regards that fever which proceeds from the obſtructed *Lochia*, and in which the breaſts may likewiſe be affected: but the milk fever is that in which the breaſts are originally concerned, and which may happen, though the *Lochia* continue to flow in ſufficient quantity; nevertheleſs, they mutually promote each other, and both are to be treated in the manner already explained; namely, by opiates,

 diluents,

diluents, and diaphoretics, in the beginning; and, theſe preſcriptions failing, the obſtructions muſt be reſolved by the antiphlogiſtic method deſcribed above. The milk fever alone, when the *Uterus* is not concerned, is not ſo dangerous, and much more eaſily relieved. Women of an healthy conſtitution, who ſuckle their own children, have good nipples, and whoſe milk comes freely, are ſeldom or never ſubject to this diſorder; which is more incident to thoſe who do not give ſuck, and neglect to prevent the ſecretion in time; or when the milk is ſecreted, take no meaſures for emptying their breaſts. This fever likewiſe happens to women who try too ſoon to ſuckle, and continue their efforts too long at one time; by which means the nipples, and conſequently the breaſts, are often inflamed, ſwelled, and obſtructed.

In order to prevent too great a turgency in the veſſels of the breaſts, and the ſecretion of milk, in thoſe women who do not chooſe to ſuckle, it will be proper to make external application of thoſe things which, by their preſſure and repercuſſive force, will hinder the blood from flowing in too great quantity

to

to this part, which is now more yielding than at any other time: for this purpoſe, let the breaſts be covered with *Emp. de minio*, *Diapalma*, or *Emp. ſimp.* ſpread upon linnen, or cloths dipped in camphorated ſpirits, be frequently applied to theſe parts and the armpits; while the patient's diet and drink is of the lighteſt kind, and given in ſmall quantities. Notwithſtanding theſe precautions, a turgency commonly begins about the third day; but by reſt, moderate ſweating, and the uſe of theſe applications, the tenſion and pain will ſubſide about the fifth or ſixth day, eſpecially if the milk runs out at the nipples: but if the woman catches cold, or is of a full habit of body, and not very abſtemious, the tenſion and pain increaſing, will bring on a cold ſhivering, ſucceeded by a fever; which may obſtruct the other excretions, as well as thoſe of the breaſt.

In this caſe, the ſudorificks above recommended, muſt be preſcribed, and if a plentiful ſweat enſues, the patient will be relieved; at the ſame time the milk muſt be extracted from her breaſts, by ſucking with the mouth or glaſſes: ſhould theſe methods fail, and the fever increaſe, ſhe ought to be blooded in the arm; and inſtead of the external applications hitherto uſed, emollient liniments and cataplaſms muſt be ſubſtituted, in order to ſoften and relax. If, in ſpite of theſe endeavours, the fever proceeds for ſome days, the patient is frequently relieved by critical ſweats, a large diſcharge from the *Uterus*, miliary eruptions, or looſe ſtools mixed with milk, which is curdled in the inteſtines: but ſhould none of theſe evacuations happen, and the inflammation continue with increaſing violence, there is danger of an impoſthume, which is to be brought to maturity, and managed like other inflammatory tumours; and no aſtringents ought to be applied, leſt they ſhould produce ſchirrous ſwellings in the glands.

As the criſis of this fever, as well as of that laſt deſcribed, often conſiſts in miliary eruptions over the whole ſurface of the body, but particularly on the neck and breaſts, by which the fever is carried off, nothing ought to be given, which will either greatly increaſe or diminiſh the circulating force; but ſuch only as will keep out the eruptions. But if, not-

with-

withſtanding theſe eruptions, the fever, inſtead of abating, is augmented, it will be neceſſary to diminiſh its force, and prevent its increaſe, by thoſe evacuations we have mentioned above. On the contrary, ſhould the pulſe ſink, the eruptions begin to retreat inwardly, and the morbific matter be in danger of falling upon the *Viſcera*, we muſt endeavour to keep them out, by ſuch opiates and ſudorific medicines as we have already preſcribed in obſtructions of the *Lochia*. On this ſubject Sir *David Hamilton* and *Hoffman* may be conſulted.

SECT. VII.

Of the PROLAPSUS VAGINÆ, RECTI ET UTERI.

WHEN the head of the child is long retained about the middle of the *Vagina*, the lower part of that ſheath ſometimes ſwells; and as the head comes farther down, is puſhed out at the *Os externum*, occaſioning great difficulty in delivering the woman: ſometimes, alſo, the lower part of the *Rectum* is protruded through the *Sphincter ani*, eſpecially if the patient is troubled with the inward piles. The cure of both theſe complaints, conſiſts in reducing the *Prolapſus*: if this cannot be done immediately in the laſt, on account of the ſwelling of the protruded part, emollient fomentations and pultices muſt be uſed, in order to remove the inflammation. When it is reduced, the woman muſt be confined more than uſual to her bed; and if the part falls down again, in conſequence of her ſtraining at ſtool, or in making water, it muſt be reduced occaſionally, and as ſhe recovers ſtrength, the complaint will in all probability vaniſh: otherwiſe, aſtringent fumigations or fomentations muſt be uſed. If the diſorder be of long duration, peſſaries, adapted to the part, whether *Vagina* or *Rectum*, muſt be applied.

A *Prolapſus uteri* may happen from the ſame cauſes, or from any thing that will too much relax the ligaments and *Peritoneum*, by which the womb is ſuſpended; ſuch as, an inveterate *Fluor albus*, that by its long continuance and great diſcharge, weakens the woman, and all theſe parts.

This

This misfortune, when it proceeds from labour, does not appear till after delivery, when the *Uterus* is contracted to its ſmalleſt ſize; nay, not for ſeveral weeks or months after that period, until, by its weight, the *Os externum* is gradually ſtretched wider and wider, ſo as to allow the womb to ſlip through it; and in this caſe, it deſcends covered with the *Vagina*, that comes down along with it, and hangs between the thighs: though the *Os tincæ* only can be perceived on account of this covering, the ſhape and ſubſtance of the *Uterus* may be eaſily diſtinguiſhed.

As this *Prolapſus* comes on gradually, the woman of herſelf can (for the moſt part) reduce and keep it up, while in bed; but when ſhe riſes and walks, it will fall down again. When the complaint is not of long ſtanding, and the womb does not come altogether through the *Os externum*, the patient may be cured by aſtringent injections; and in the next pregnancy, when the upper part of the *Uterus* is diſtended, ſo as to fill the *Pelvis*, and riſe above its brim, the *Os internum* will be raiſed higher in the *Vagina*;

and after delivery, if the woman is confined to her bed for twenty or thirty days, the ligaments generally contract, ſo as to keep up the womb, and prevent any future *Prolapſus:* but when the complaint is of long continuance; when the *Uterus* and *Vagina* deſcend quite through the *Os externum*, and by the friction in walking, occaſioned by the *Vagina*'s rubbing againſt the thighs and the *Os uteri*, upon the cloaths that are uſed for ſupporting it, an inflammation, excoriation, and ulceration, is produced, inviting a greater flux of fluids to the part: theſe ſymptoms, joined with a *Fluor albus* from the inſide of the *Uterus*, deſtroy the hope of a ſecond impregnation, or cure by injections, and we can only promiſe to palliate the diſeaſe, by reducing the *Uterus*, and keeping it up with a peſſary; by which means uſed for a length of time, perhaps the parts will recover their tone, and the diſeaſe be radically cured.

If the *Uterus* be ſo much inflamed, that it cannot be reduced, general evacuations muſt be preſcribed, fomentations and pultices applied, in order to diminiſh its bulk, ſo as that it may be replaced: for this complaint,

dif-

different kinds of peſſaries have been uſed; ſome of a globular form, others that open with a ſpring, as deſcribed in the medical eſſays of *Edinburgh*. But thoſe moſt in uſe are of a flat form, with a little hole in the middle, and made of cork waxed over, ivory, box, ebony, lignum vitæ, of a triangular, quadrangular, oval, or circular ſhape. Thoſe that are circular ſeem beſt to anſwer the intention, becauſe we can more eaſily introduce a large one of that, than of any other figure; it lies more commodiouſly in the *Vagina*, and as it always tilts a little upwards and downwards, never hinders the paſſage of the urine or *Fæces*: theſe inſtruments, however, ought to be larger or ſmaller, according to the laxity or rigidity of the *Os externum*.

There is a peſſary lately invented at *Paris*, which hath an advantage over all others; becauſe the woman can introduce it in the morning, and take it out at night: it is ſupported and kept in the *Vagina* by a ſmall ſtalk, the lower end of which forms a little ball that moves in a ſocket; this ſocket is furniſhed with ſtraps, which are tied to a

belt

belt that surrounds the patient's body. This pessary is extremely well calculated for those who are in an easy way of life; but the other kind is best adapted to hard working women, who have not time or conveniency to fix or mend the bandage when it wants repair.

SECT. VIII.

Of the Evacuations necessary at the End of the Month after Delivery.

THOSE who have had a sufficient discharge of the *Lochia*, plenty of milk, and suckle their own children, commonly recover with ease; and as the superfluous fluids of the body are drained off at the nipples, seldom require evacuations at the end of the month: but if there are any complaints from fullness, such as pains and stitches, after the twentieth day, some blood ought to be taken from the arm, and the belly gently opened by frequent glysters, or repeated doses of laxative medicines.

If the patient has tolerably recovered, the milk having been at first sucked or discharged from the nipples, and afterwards discussed, no evacuations are neceſſary before the third or fourth week; and ſometimes not till after the firſt flowing of the *Menſes*, which commonly happens about the fifth week: if they do not appear within that time, gentle evacuations muſt be preſcribed to carry off the *Plethora*, and bring down the *Catamenia*.

CHAP. II.

Of the Management of new-born Children, with the Diſeaſes to which they are ſubject.

SECT. I.

Of waſhing and dreſſing the Child.

THE child being delivered, the navel-ſtring tied and cut, a warm cloth or flannel cap put on its head, and its body wrapped in a warm receiver, it may be given to the nurſe, or an aſſiſtant, in order to be waſhed clean from that ſcarf, which ſometimes covers the whole ſcurf-ſkin, and is particularly found upon the hairy ſcalp, under the

the arm-pits, and in the groins. This ablution is commonly performed with warm water, mixed with a ſmall quantity of *Hungary* water, wine, or ale, in which a little pomatum, or freſh butter, hath been diſſolved. This compoſition cleans all the ſurface, and the oily part, by mixing with, and attenuating the *Mucus*, prepares it for the linnen cloth, which dries and wipes off the whole: nevertheleſs, milk and water, or ſoap and water, is preferable to this mixture.

In laborious or præternatural caſes, when conſiderable force hath been uſed in delivering the child, the whole body ought to be examined; and if there is any mark or contuſion, on the head, it will diſappear, if anointed with pomatum, and gently rubbed or chafed with the accoucheur's hand: if any limb is diſlocated or broke, it ought to be reduced immediately: luxations, though they ſeldom happen, are more incident to the ſhoulder than to any other part, the *Humerus* being eaſily diſlocated, and as eaſily reduced. The bones of the arm and thigh are more ſubject to fractures than any other of the extremities: the firſt is eaſily cured, be-

becauſe the limb can be kept from being moved; but a fracture in the thigh bone is a much more troubleſome caſe, becauſe, over and above the difficulty of keeping the bones in a proper ſituation, the part is often neceſſarily moved in cleaning the child. In this caſe, the beſt method is, to keep the child lying on one ſide, after the thigh hath been ſecured by proper bandage, ſo that the nurſe may change the cloth without moving the part; and to lie upon bolſters or pillows, raiſed above the wet nurſe, that it may ſuck with greater freedom: if any of the bones are bent, they may be brought into their proper form, by a ſlow, gentle, and proper reſiſtance.

The navel-ſtring muſt be wrapped in a ſoft, linnen rag, and folded up on the belly, over which is to be laid a thick compreſs, kept moderately tight with a bandage commonly called a belly-band. This compreſſion muſt be continued for ſome time, in order to prevent an *Exomphalus*, or rupture, at the navel; and kept tighter and longer on children that are addicted to crying, than on thoſe that are ſtill and quiet: yet not ſo tight

as

as to be uneaſy to the child, and the bandage muſt be looſened and the part examined, every ſecond day. The navel-ſtring ſhrinks, dries, and about the ſixth or ſeventh day, commonly drops off from the belly; though not at the ligature, as ſome people have imagined. This being ſeparated, a pledget of dry lint muſt be applied to the navel, and over it, the thick compreſs and bandage, to be continued ſeveral weeks, for the purpoſe mentioned above.

During the time of waſhing and dreſſing the child, it ought to be kept moderately warm, eſpecially in the head and breaſt, that the cold air may not obſtruct perſpiration: the head and body ought alſo to be kept tolerably tight with the cloaths, for the convenience of handling, and to prevent its catching cold, eſpecially if the child be weakly; but if it is vigorous and full grown, it cannot be too looſely cloathed, becauſe the brain, *Thorax*, and *Abdomen*, ſuffer by too great compreſſion. The cloathing of new-born children ought alſo to be ſuitable to the ſeaſon of the year, and the nature of the weather; the extremes of cold and heat being avoided,

avoided, as equally hurtful and dangerous. Inſtead of the many ſuperfluous inventions of nurſes, and thoſe who make cloaths for children, with a view to make an expenſive and pompous appearance, the dreſs ought to be contrived with all imaginable ſimplicity: the child being waſhed, the navel-ſtring ſecured, and the head covered with a linnen or woollen cap, as already directed, a ſhirt and waiſtcoat may be put upon the body, and over it a flannel ſkirt or petticoat, open before, with a broad head-band, as commonly uſed, or rather a waiſtcoat joined to it, ſo as that they can be put on at once: this ought to be rather tied than pinned before, and, inſtead of two or more blankets, may be covered with a flannel or fuſtian gown; while the head is accommodated with another cap, adorned with as much finery as the tire-woman ſhall think proper to beſtow.

In ſhort, the principal aim in this point is to keep the child's head and body neither too tight nor too ſlovenly, too hot nor too cold; that it may be warm, though not over-heated, and eaſy, though not too looſe; that reſpiration may be full and large; that the brain

may

may ſuffer no compreſſion; and that, while the child is awake, the legs may be at liberty; to reject all unneceſſary rollers, croſs-cloths, neckcloths, and blankets; and to uſe as few pins as poſſible, and thoſe that are abſolutely neceſſary, with the utmoſt caution.

SECT. II.

How to manage when any of the common paſſages are locked up, or the tongue tied.

WHEN the child cannot make water, becauſe the paſſage is filled up with *Mucus*; after having unſucceſsfully practiſed the common methods of holding the belly near the fire, and rubbing the parts with *Ol. Rutæ*, &c. we muſt introduce a probe, or very ſmall catheter, along the *Urethra*, into the bladder; an operation much more eaſily performed in female than in male children.

In boys, the prepuce alone is ſometimes imperforated; in which caſe, an opening is eaſily made: but if there is no paſſage in the *Urethra*, or even through the whole length of the *Glans*, all that can be done is to make an opening, with a lancet or biſtory, near the

the mouth or ſphincter of the bladder, in the lower part of the *Urethra*; where the urine being obſtructed, puſhes out the parts in form of a tumour: or if no ſuch tumefaction appears, to perforate the bladder above the *Pubis*, with a trocar: this, however, is a wretched and ineffectual expedient, and the other can but at beſt lengthen out a miſerable life. If the *Anus* is imperforated, and the *Fæces* protrude the parts; or if it be covered with a thin membrane, and a bluiſh or livid ſpot appears, the puncture and inciſion commonly ſucceed; but when the *Rectum* is altogether wanting, or impervious for a conſiderable way, the ſucceſs of the operation is very uncertain: nevertheleſs, it ought to be tried, by making an artificial *Anus*, with a biſtory, remembering the courſe of the *Rectum*, and the entry in both ſexes. For further information on this ſubject, *Mauriceau*'s and *Savoiard*'s obſervations, and the memoirs of the academy of ſurgeons, may be conſulted.

In female children, there is a thin membrane, in form of a creſcent, called the *Hymen*, that covers the lower part of the orifice of the *Vagina*, and is rent in the firſt coition. The middle of it is ſometimes attached to the lower part of the *Meatus urinarius*, and on each ſide of the bridge is a ſmall opening, that will only admit the end of a probe, though it is ſufficient for the diſcharge of the *Menſes*. This obſtruction is commonly unknown till marriage, and hath often proved fatal to the unfortunate woman, who had concealed it through exceſs of modeſty, and afterwards ſunk into a deep melancholy, which coſt her her life; rather than ſubmit to inſpection, and the eaſy cure of having the attachment ſnipt with a pair of ſciſſars. On this conſideration, *Savoiard* adviſes all accoucheurs to inſpect this part in every female child they deliver; and if there ſhould be ſuch a defect, remedy it during her childhood: or if the entry is wholly covered with the membrane, make a ſufficient perforation; which will prevent great pain and tenſion in their riper years, when the *Menſes* being denied paſſage, would accumulate every month, and at laſt puſh out this and the neighbouring parts in form of a large tumour, the

cauſe

cauſe of which is generally unknown, until it be opened.

Sometimes, a thin membrane riſing from the under part of the mouth, ſtretches almoſt to the tip of the tongue, bracing it down, ſo as to hinder the child from taking hold of the nipple, and ſucking. This diſorder, which is called tongue-tying, is eaſily remedied by introducing the fore finger into the child's mouth, raiſing up the tongue, and ſnipping the bridle with a pair of ſciſſars.

If, inſtead of a thin membrane, the tongue is confined by a thick, fleſhy ſubſtance, the ſafeſt method is, to direct the nurſe to ſtretch it frequently and gently with her finger; or if it appears like a ſoft *Fungus*, to touch it frequently and cautiouſly with lunar cauſtick, or *Roman* vitriol: but we ought to take care that we are not deceived by an inflammation that ſometimes happens in the birth, from the accoucheur's helping the head along with his finger in the child's mouth.

SECT. III.

Of Mould-ſhot Heads, Contuſions, and Excoriations.

IN laborious and lingering labours, the child's head is often long confined, and ſo compreſſed in the *Pelvis*, that the bones of the upper part of the *Cranium* are ſqueezed together, and ride over one another, in different manners, according as the head preſented. If the *Oſſa parietalia* riſe over the *Os Frontis*, the caſe is called the mould-ſhot; if over the *Occiput*, it goes by the name of the horſe-ſhoe mould. When the *Fontanelle* preſents, (though this is ſeldom the caſe) and is puſhed down, the form of the head is raiſed up in the ſhape of an hog's back; whereas, in the former caſe, the *Vertex* or crown of the head preſented, and the whole was turned from a round to a very long figure. If the head is kept long in the *Pelvis*, and the child not deſtroyed by the compreſſion of the brain, either before or ſoon after delivery, it commonly retains more or leſs of the ſhape acquired in that ſituation,

ac-

according to the ſtrength or weakneſs of the child. When the bones begin to ride over one another in this manner, the hairy ſcalp is felt lax and wrinkled; but, by the long preſſure and obſtructions of the circulating fluids, it gradually ſwells, and forms a large tumour.

In theſe caſes, when the child is delivered, we ought to allow the navel ſtring, at cutting, to bleed from one to two or three ſpoonfuls, eſpecially if the infant be vigorous and full grown; and to provoke it by whipping and ſtimulating: for the more it cries, the ſooner and better are the bones of the *Cranium* forced outwards into their natural ſituation: or if the head hath not been long compreſſed, and is not much inflamed, we can ſometimes, with our hands, reduce it into its priſtine ſhape. The *Meconium* ought alſo to be purged off as ſoon as poſſible, to give freer ſcope to the circulating fluids in the *Abdomen*, and make a revulſion from the ſurcharged and compreſſed brain. This may be effected with ſuppoſitories, glyſters, repeated doſes of *Ol. Amygdal. d.* mixed with

 Pulv.

Pulv. Rhababari. or *De Althæa,* or *Syr. de Cichoreo, cum Rheo.*

If the child is ſeized with convulſions ſoon after delivery, in conſequence of this compreſſion, and the veſſels of the navel-ſtring have not been allowed to bleed, the jugular vein ought immediately to be opened, and from one to two ounces of blood taken away; an operation eaſily performed in young children: the urine and *Meconium* muſt be diſcharged, and a ſmall bliſter applied between the *Scapulæ.* When the ſcalp is bruiſed, inflamed, or ſwelled, let it be anointed, or embrocated, with a mixture of *Ol. Chamomel. Acet.* and *Spt. Vin. Camphorat.* and *Cerates,* and pultices applied to the parts.

If the tumefaction is large, and we feel a conſiderable fluctuation of extravaſated fluids, which cannot be taken up by the abſorbent veſſels, aſſiſted with thoſe applications, the tumour muſt be opened; though generally there is no occaſion for a large inciſion, becauſe after the fluid is once diſcharged, the hollow ſcalp, by gentle preſſure, is more eaſily joined in children than in older ſubjects.

When

When the head is miſhapen, it ſhould not be bound or preſſed, but left lax and eaſy; leſt, the brain being compreſſed, convulſions ſhould enſue.

The body of the child is ſometimes covered all over with little red ſpots, called the red gum, and commonly proceeding from the coſtiveneſs of the child, when the *Meconium* hath not been ſufficiently purged off at firſt. And here it will not be improper to obſerve, that as the whole tract of the *Colon* is filled with this viſcid excrement, which hath been gradually accumulated for a conſiderable time; and as the ſmall inteſtines, ſtomach and gullet are lined with a glary fluid or *Mucus*, the child ought to take no other nouriſhment than pap as thin as whey, to dilute this fluid, for the firſt two days; or indeed, till it ſucks the mother's milk, which begins to be ſecreted about the third day, and is at firſt ſufficiently purgative to diſcharge theſe humours; and better adapted for the purpoſe than any artificial purge.

If the mother's milk cannot be had, a nurſe lately delivered is to be found; and if the purgative quality of her milk is decreaſed, ſhe muſt be ordered to take repeated ſmall doſes of manna or lenitive electuary; by which it will recover its former virtue, and the child be ſufficiently purged.

If the child is brought up by hand, the food ought to imitate, as near as poſſible, the mother's milk: let it conſiſt of loaf-bread and water, boiled up together, in form of panada, and mixed with the ſame quantity of new cow's milk; and ſometimes with the broth of fowl or mutton. When the child is coſtive, two drachms of manna, or from two to four grains of rhubarb, may be given: and when the ſtools are green and curdled, it will be proper to abſorb the prevailing acid with the teſtaceous powders; ſuch as the *Chel. Cancror. ſimp.* or *Teſt. Oſtrear*, given from the quantity of ten grains to a ſcruple: and for this purpoſe, the *Magneſia alba* is recommended, from one to two drachms a day, as being both opening and abſorbent. The red gum may likewiſe proceed from the officiouſneſs of the nurſe, by which the ſcurf ſkin hath been abraded, or rubbed off; in which caſe, the child muſt be bathed in warm milk, and the parts ſoftened with po-

matum;

matum: the ſame bath may be alſo uſed daily in the other kind, and the belly kept open with the aforementioned medicines; with which, ſome ſyrup, tincture, or powder of rhubarb, may be mixed, or given by itſelf, if the ſtools are of a greeniſh hue.

Excoriations behind the ears, in the neck and groin of the child, are ſometimes, indeed, unavoidable in fat and groſs habits; but moſt commonly proceed from the careleſsneſs of the nurſe, who neglects to waſh and keep the parts clean: they are, however, eaſily dried up and healed, with *Unguent. Alb. Pulv. e Ceruſſa*, or fuller's earth. Yet we ought to be cautious in applying drying medicines behind the ears, becauſe a diſcharge in that part frequently prevents worſe diſeaſes.

SECT. IV.

Of the APTHA.

THE *Aptha*, or thruſh, is a diſeaſe to which new-born children are frequently ſubject, and is often dangerous, when neglected at the beginning. This diſeaſe pro-

proceeds from weakneſs and laxity of the contracting force of the ſtomach and inteſtines, by which the aceſcent food is not digeſted; and from a defect in the neceſſary ſecretion of bile, with which it ought to be mixed. This prevailing acid in the *Primæ viæ*, produces gripings and looſe green ſtools, that weaken the child more and more, deprive it of its proper nouriſhment and reſt, and occaſion a fever from inanition and irritation. The ſmalleſt veſſels at the mouths of the excretory ducts in the mouth, gullet, ſtomach and inteſtines, are obſtructed and ulcerated in conſequence of the child's weakneſs and acrimonious vomitings, belchings, and ſtools, and little foul ulcers are formed.

Theſe firſt appear in ſmall white ſpecks on the lips, mouth, tongue, and at the fundament: they gradually increaſe in thickneſs and extent; adopt a yellow colour, which in the progreſs of the diſtemper becomes duſkiſh, and the watry ſtools (called the watry gripes) become more frequent. The whole inner ſurface of the inteſtines being thus ulcerated and obſtructed, no nouriſhment enters the lacteal veſſels; ſo that the weakneſs and diſ-

diſeaſe are increaſed, the milk and pap which are taken in at the mouth, paſſes off curdled and green, the child is more and more enfeebled, and the brown colour of the *Aptha* declares a mortification, and death at hand. Sometimes, however, the *Apthæ* are unattended by the watry ſtools; and ſometimes, theſe laſt are unaccompanied with the *Aptha*.

In order to prevent this fatal cataſtrophe, at the firſt appearance of the diſorder, we ought to preſcribe repeated doſes of teſtaceous powders, to abſorb and ſweeten the predominant acid in the ſtomach, giving them from ten to twenty grains in the pap, twice or three times a day; and on every third night, from three to five grains of the *Pulv. Rhei, Julap. e Creta*; oily and anodyne glyſters, with epithems to the ſtomach, may alſo be adminiſtred. When theſe, and every other preſcription fail, the child, if not much weakened, is ſometimes cured by a gentle vomit, conſiſting of *Pulv. Ipecacuan.* gr. I. given in a ſpoonful of barley-water, and repeated two or three times, at the interval of half an hour between each. When the child is much enfeebled, the *Oleo-Saccharum Cinnamomi*,

namomi, or *Anisi*, mixed with the pap, is ſometimes ſerviceable. If the milk is either too purgative or binding, the nurſe ſhould be changed, or take proper medicines to alter its quality: or if the child has been brought up by hand, woman's milk may be given on this occaſion, together with weak broths; but if the child cannot ſuck, the milk of cows, mares, or aſſes, may be ſubſtituted in its room, diluted with barley-water.

SECT. V.

Of Teething.

CHILDREN commonly begin to breed their fore teeth about the ſeventh, and ſometimes not before the ninth month; nay, in ſome, the period is ſtill later. Thoſe who are healthy and lax in their bellies, undergo dentition eaſier than ſuch as are of a contrary conſtitution. When the teeth ſhoot from the ſockets, and their ſharp points begin to work their way through the *Perioſteum* and gums, they frequently produce great pain and inflammation, which, if they continue violent, bring on feveriſh ſymptoms and convulſions,

vulſions, that often prove fatal. In order to prevent theſe misfortunes, the ſwelled gum may, at firſt, be cut down to the tooth, with a biſtory or fleam; by which means the patient is often relieved immediately: but if the child is ſtrong, the pulſe quick, the ſkin hot and dry, bleeding at the jugular will be alſo neceſſary, and the belly muſt be kept open with repeated glyſters. On the other hand, if the child is low, ſunk, and emaciated, repeated doſes of *Spt. C. C. Tinct. Fuligin.* and the like, may be preſcribed; and bliſters applied to the back, or behind the ears.

CHAP.

CHAP. III.

Of the requiſite Qualifications of Accoucheurs, Midwives, Nurſes who attend lying-in women, and wet and dry Nurſes for Children.

SECT. I.

Of the ACCOUCHEUR.

THOSE who intend to practice midwifery, ought firſt of all to make themſelves maſters of anatomy, and acquire a competent knowledge in ſurgery and phyſick; becauſe of their connexions with the obſtetric art, if not always, at leaſt in many caſes. He ought to take the beſt opportunities he can find, of being well inſtructed; and of practiſing under a maſter, before he attempts to deliver by himſelf.

In order to acquire a more perfect idea of the art, he ought to perform with his own hands upon proper machines, contrived to convey a juſt notion of all the difficulties to be met with in every kind of labour; by which means, he will learn how to uſe the forceps and crotchets with more dexterity, be accuſtomed to the turning of children, and conſequently the more capable of acquitting himſelf in troubleſome caſes, that may happen to him when he comes to practiſe among women: he ſhould alſo embrace every occaſion of being preſent at real labours, and indeed of acquiring every qualification that may be neceſſary or convenient for him in the future exerciſe of his profeſſion: but over and above the advantages of education, he ought to be endued with a natural ſagacity, reſolution, and prudence; together with that humanity which adorns the owner, and never fails of being agreeable to the diſtreſſed patient: in conſequence of this virtue, he will aſſiſt the poor as well as the rich, behaving always with charity and compaſſion. He ought to act and ſpeak with the utmoſt delicacy of decorum, and never violate the truſt repoſed in him, ſo as to harbour the leaſt immoral or indecent deſign; but demean himſelf in all reſpects ſuitable to the dignity of his profeſſion.

SECT. II.

Of the MIDWIFE.

A Midwife, though ſhe can hardly be ſuppoſed miſtreſs of all theſe qualifications, ought to be a decent, ſenſible woman, of a middle age, able to bear fatigue; ſhe ought to be perfectly well inſtructed with regard to the bones of the *Pelvis*, with all the contained parts, comprehending thoſe that are ſubſervient to generation; ſhe ought to be well ſkill'd in the method of touching pregnant women, and know in what manner the womb ſtretches, together with the ſituation of all the abdominal *Viſcera*; ſhe ought to be perfectly miſtreſs of the art of examination in time of labour, together with all the different kinds of labour, whether natural or præternatural, and the methods of delivering the *Placenta*; ſhe ought to live in friendſhip with other women of the ſame profeſſion, contending with them in nothing but in knowledge, ſobriety, diligence, and patience; ſhe ought to void all reflections upon men practitioners, and when ſhe finds her-

herſelf difficulted, candidly have recourſe to their aſſiſtance: on the other hand, this confidence ought to be encouraged by the man, who, when called, inſtead of openly condemning her method of practice, (even though it ſhould be erroneous) ought to make allowance for the weakneſs of the ſex, and rectify what is amiſs, without expoſing her miſtakes. This conduct will as effectually conduce to the welfare of the patient, and operate as a ſilent rebuke upon the conviction of the midwife; who finding herſelf treated ſo tenderly, will be more apt to call for neceſſary aſſiſtance on future occaſions, and to conſider the accoucheur as a man of honour, and a real friend. Theſe gentle methods will prevent that mutual calumny and abuſe which too often prevail among the male and female practitioners, and redound to the advantage of both: for, no accoucheur is ſo perfect, but that he may err ſometimes; and on ſuch occaſions, he muſt expect to meet with retaliation from thoſe midwives whom he may have roughly uſed.

SECT. III.

Of NURSES *in general.*

NURSES, as well as midwives, ought to be of a middle age, ſober, patient, and diſcreet, able to bear fatigue and watching, free from external deformity, cutaneous eruptions and inward complaints, that may be troubleſome or infectious.

NUMB. I.

NURSES that attend lying-in women, ought to have provided, and in order, every thing that may be neceſſary for the woman, accoucheur, midwife, and child; ſuch as linnen and cloaths, well aired and warm, for the woman and the bed, which ſhe muſt know how to prepare when there is occaſion; together with nutmeg, ſugar, ſpirit of hartſhorn, vinegar, *Hungary* water, white or brown caudle ready made, and a glyſter-pipe fitted. For the uſe of the accoucheur, ſhe muſt hang a doubled ſheet over the bed ſide, and prepare warm cloaths, pomatum, thread, warm and cold water, and two hand-baſins; and

and for dreſſing the child, ſhe muſt keep the cloaths warm and in good order. After delivery, her buſineſs is to tend the mother and child with the utmoſt care, and follow the directions given to her, relating to the management of each.

That the mother herſelf ſhould give ſuck, would certainly be moſt conducive to her own recovery, as well as to the health of the child; but when this is inconvenient, or impracticable, from her weakneſs, or circumſtances in life, a wet nurſe ought to be hired, poſſeſſed of the qualifications above deſcribed, as well as of thoſe that follow.

NUMB. II.

THE younger the milk is, the better will it agree with the age of the infant. The nurſe is more valuable after having brought forth her ſecond child, than after her firſt; becauſe ſhe is endued with more knowledge and experience touching the management of children. She ought to have good nipples, with a ſufficient quantity of good milk: the abundance or ſcantineſs of the ſecretion may be diſtinguiſhed by the appearance of her own child; and the quality may be aſcertained by examining the milk, which ſhe may be ordered to pour into a wine glaſs, about two or three hours after ſhe hath eaten and drank, and ſuckled her own child. If, when falling in a ſingle drop upon the nail, it runs off immediately, the milk is too thin; if the drop ſtands in a round globe, it is too thick; but when the drop remains in a flattened form, the milk is judged to be of a right conſiſtence: in a word, it may be as well diſtinguiſhed by its opacity or tranſparency, when it is daſhed up on the ſide of the glaſs: beſides, it ought to be ſweet to the taſte, and in colour inclining to blue rather than to yellow. Red-hair'd women, or ſuch as are very fair and delicate, are commonly objected to in the quality of nurſes; but this maxim is not without exceptions: and on this ſubject, *Boerhaave*'s inſtitutes, with *Haller*'s commentary, may be conſulted.

Although it is certainly moſt natural for children to ſuck, it may be ſometimes neceſſary to bring them up by hand; that is, nouriſh them with pap: becauſe proper wet nurſes cannot always be found, and many chil-

children have ſuffered by ſucking diſeaſed women. Some can never be brought to ſuck, although they have no apparent hinderance; and others are prevented by ſome ſwelling or diſorder about the mouth or throat.

NUMB. III.

UPON ſuch occaſions, we muſt chooſe an elderly woman properly qualified for the taſk, and well accuſtomed to the duties of a dry nurſe. The food (as we have formerly obſerved) ought to be light and ſimple, in quality reſembling, as nearly as poſſible, the mother's milk; ſuch as thin panada, mixed with cow's milk, and ſweetened with ſugar: or ſhould the child be coſtive, inſtead of ſugar, honey or manna may be uſed. If there is any reaſon to believe, that the loaf-bread or biſcuit is made of flour which hath been mixed with allum, for the ſake of the colour, the common panada ought in this caſe to be laid aſide, in favour of thick water-gruel, mixed with milk, and ſweetened as above.

Some children thrive very well on this diet, but when it is neither agreeable to their palates, nor nouriſhing, a wet nurſe muſt be procured, before the child is too much emaciated and exhauſted; and if it can ſuck, the good effects of the milk will ſoon be manifeſt. But for further information, on this head, the reader may conſult Dr. *Cadogan*'s letter on the nurſing of children.

F I N I S.

ADVERTISEMENT.

DOCTOR *Smellie* having, with great care and expence, employed Mr. *Riemſdyk* to draw anatomical figures, as large as the human ſubjects themſelves, for the uſe of thoſe who attend his lectures, and in order to illuſtrate his theory and practice of midwifery; and being deſirous to render his drawings of more extenſive and general uſe, by cauſing them to be engraved by able artiſts, a deſign which cannot be put in execution without a conſiderable expence; he propoſes to publiſh the whole ſet by ſubſcription, in the following manner:

I.

The work will conſiſt of twenty-ſix plates, of about 18 inches by 12.

ADVERTISEMENT.

II.

A full and diſtinct explanation of each plate will be printed on a large ſheet, of the ſame ſize with the figures, that they may be bound up together. For the uſe of foreigners, there will alſo be an explanation printed in *Latin*, and a liſt of the ſubſcribers ſhall be publiſhed, if deſired.

III.

The price to ſubſcribers will be two guineas, one to be paid at the time of ſubſcribing, and the other at the delivery of the prints, with their explanations.

IV.

The drawings will be put into the hands of the beſt engravers, as ſoon as a number of ſubſcriptions are received ſufficient to defray the expence of the work, which will be executed with as great diſpatch as ſhall be conſiſtent with the nature and accuracy of the performance.

PLATE I.

ADVERTISEMENT.

PLATE I.

Repreſents the bones of a well formed *Pelvis*, in a front view.

2d. A ſide view of the ſame. This and the former, deſigned to aſcertain the width, depth and form of the inſide.

3d. The front view of a diſtorted *Pelvis*.

4th, A view of the external parts, in order to exhibit the ſituation and appearance of the *Os Externum*, *Anus*, *Coccyx*, and the lower ends of the *Iſchia*.

5th, Repreſents the internal parts, in three figures. FIG. I. Exhibits a front view of the internal parts of a young woman in the firſt month of her firſt pregnancy; namely, the *Uterus* in the natural ſituation hanging down in the *Vagina*. FIG. 2. Repreſents a ſide view of the ſame parts, in a woman of a middle age, who hath had children; one half cut off lengthways. FIG. 3. Gives a front view of the *Uterus* cut open, to ſhew the inſide, and the embryo appearing through the *Amnios*, the *Uterus* being as large as that in FIG. 2. and in a ſecond pregnancy.

6th

6th, Containing 2 Figures.

FIG. 1. Reprefents the *Uterus* in the fecond or third month of the firft pregnancy, with the *Embryo* inclofed, raifed up, as in touching, to fhew the *Vagina* ftretched in length. FIG. 2. Exhibits the fame in the fourth or fifth month, the womb filling the upper part of the *Pelvis*, the neck fhortened, and towards the lower part of the *Vagina*.

7th, Reprefents the *Uterus* in the fixth or feventh month, refting on the brim of the *Pelvis*, with the *Fœtus* contained; the neck ftill fhorter than in the former figure.

8th, Reprefents the *Uterus* in the eighth or ninth month; the *Fœtus* intangled in the *Funis*, and the head prefenting, part of the *Placenta* and membranes at the back part of the *Uterus*, the neck of which is totally ftretched, and the *Os internum* larger and fofter than in the former plate.

9th, Exhibits the reprefentation of twins at the full time, the loweft prefenting with the head; the breech of the other being

turned

turned downwards, and intangled in the umbilical rope, the woman in labour, and the *Os internum* a little opened.

10th, Shews the membranes dilating the *Os Uteri*, in time of a labour-pain; the surface of the *Chorion* and *Placenta* near the *Fundus*, and the lower part of the child seen through the *Amnios*, the *Chorion* being split at that place.

11th, Represents the mouth of the womb fully open, (the membranes being broke, and some part of the waters discharged) the head engaged in the upper part of the *Pelvis*, with one ear to the *Pubis*. Part of the *Funis* with an hand appearing before the head.

12th, Shews the head at the lower part of the *Pelvis*, the *Vertex* being turned below the *Pubis*, and the forehead into the concavity of the *Sacrum*. This in a side view of the *Pelvis*, the waters being wholly discharged.

13th, Represents the head in a position quite the reverse of the former, namely, a

side

ſide view, ſhewing the *Vertex* in the hollow of the *Sacrum*, and the forehead turned to the *Pubis*.

14th, Repreſents the *Vertex* dilating the *Os Externum*, and protruding the *Perinæum*, *Anus*, and neighbouring parts, in form of a large tumour.

15th contains, The repreſentation of the forceps, ſpecified by the letters *a*. *b*. a blunt hook or crotchet *c*.

16, The delineation of one blade of a larger pair of forceps bent to one ſide, *a*.

Leveret's *tire tête* altered, *b*, *c*.

A polypus forceps, *d*.

17th, Repreſents the figure of the *Arabian Impellens* and a perforator, with two hooks or arms, *a*, *b*.

Two kinds of peſſaries, *c*. *d*.

The fillet and whalebone, *e*.

The nooſe forceps, *f f*.

A woman's catheter, *g*.

A dilator, *h*.

18th, Contains the figure of *Meſnard*'s curve crotchets improved, *a*, *b*, *c*.

A pair of ſciſſars, with reſts or ſtops, *d*.

19th,

19th, Repreſents the breech of the child preſenting, the back being turned to the forepart of the *Uterus*; a knot upon the *Funis umbilicalis*.

20th, Exhibits another view of the ſame, the breech being lower down in the *Pelvis*, and the thighs towards the *Pubis*.

21ſt, Repreſents the *Fœtus* compreſſed into a round form, the arms *Funis*, and legs, preſenting in the *Vagina*.

22d, Repreſents the *Fœtus* in the ſame form, the back parts preſenting, the head, legs, and one arm being towards the fore part and *Fundus* of the womb, and the other arm in the *Vagina*.

23d, Shews the breaſt preſenting, one arm protruded to the *Os Externum*, and the other lying double in the *Vagina*; the head and feet reflected over the back, towards the *Fundus Uteri*.

24th, Shews the forehead preſenting at the brim of the *Pelvis*; the face to one ſide, and the *Fontanelle* to the other; the feet and breech to the *Fundus*, and the *Ute-*

rus

rus contracted in form of a ſheath, around the body of the child.

25th, Is a ſide view of the *Pelvis*, ſhewing the face preſenting, the chin below the *Pubis*, and the forehead in the hollow of the *Sacrum*.

26th, Repreſents a poſition the reverſe of the former; the *Fontanelle* at the *Pubis*, and the chin at the lower part of the *Sacrum*.

In each plate the child is repreſented in its own *Uterus*, the forepart of which is cut off, in order to exhibit the inſide view, together with the ſize and ſituation of the *Fœtus*.

The womb, ligaments and *Vagina*, are ſhewn in their proper ſituation and appearance, according to the time of pregnancy. Part of the bones of the *Pelvis* are removed, but their out-lines are marked ſo as to demonſtrate their ſituation, with regard to the other parts.

N. B.

ADVERTISEMENT.

N. B. Theſe prints, and the treatiſe on the theory and practice of Midwifery, together with the volume of caſes hereafter to be publiſhed, will compoſe a compleat ſyſtem of the art.